THE
ONE THING
HOLDING
YOU BACK

THE
ONE THING
HOLDING
YOU BACK

UNLEASHING *the* POWER *of* EMOTIONAL CONNECTION

RAPHAEL CUSHNIR

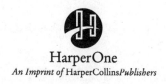

HarperOne
An Imprint of HarperCollins*Publishers*

HarperOne

The stories of emotional connection presented in this book are culled from my detailed notes gathered over the past decade. To protect client privacy, I have changed identifying details. For the purposes of clarity and instructional precision, I have also streamlined, blended, and slightly altered some of the accounts.

HarperCollins books may be purchased for educational, business, or sales promotional use. For information please write: Special Markets Department, HarperCollins Publishers, 10 East 53rd Street, New York, NY 10022.

HarperCollins Web site: http://www.harpercollins.com

HarperCollins®, 🏭®, and HarperOne™ are trademarks of HarperCollins Publishers

FIRST EDITION

Library of Congress Cataloging-in-Publication Data is available.
ISBN 978-0-06-089739-0

09 10 11 12 13   RRD(H)   10 9 8 7 6 5 4 3 2 1

For my three muses

Traci, Hazel, and Aria Belle

CONTENTS

PART FOUR

Profiles in Emotional Connection

INTRODUCTION

Everyone wants to succeed. Everyone wants more of something, whether freedom, power, love, fame, money, pleasure, peace, service, healing, growth, or change. Most people want their own unique combination of these goals. Even people who have given up hope or become willing to settle for far less still have secret visions of what their lives might look like, might feel like, if only they were different.

What about you? What do you want? If you already know the answer, if your own definition of success is perfectly clear, this book will help you achieve it. If you're uncertain, confused, or in the process of reevaluating your life vision, this book will help you refine *and* achieve it.

With life growing ever more complex for all of us, how could one book, one perspective, be equally applicable across the entire realm of human experience? The answer lies not in how each of us is different, but in what we all share.

One of the things we all share is emotion. The same range and capacity for emotion is present in every single person. Emotional neurons are firing constantly in our brains, and emotional neuropeptides are cascading similarly through our bodies. This electrochemical dance occurs from the moment we're born till the moment we die. It's as much at play in the private gaze of two lovers as it is in the most sweeping events of human history. Scientists have demonstrated that the same basic emotions of fear, anger, sadness, and joy produce facial expressions recognizable across divisions of race, class, religion, and culture. In all our feverish activity, it's been said, we're either running toward an emotion or away from one.

This running away from emotions is something else we all share. Depending on context, it may be known as repression, denial, resistance, or stoicism. Part of it is natural and ingrained—we're designed to avoid what we don't like or don't want. Part of it is beneficial—many responsibilities require that we temporarily stave off our emotions in order to focus on the task at hand. But the biggest part of it is learned, and that's where we get into trouble.

Almost everything we learn about feeling and not feeling emotions is unspoken. We pick it up in childhood by observing, and then mimicking, the behavior of those around us. This happens mostly at an unconscious level and is mostly negative.

I've had this confirmed at virtually every seminar and workshop I've ever led. Early on, I ask the participants to raise their hands if they received a sound education from their parents in how to experience and understand emotions. No hands go up. Then I ask if such an education was provided at school or religious institutions. Again, no hands. Peer group? Forget about it.

So here, in a nutshell, is our emotional predicament: when it comes to this crucial, unavoidable, and often confounding aspect of our lives, we're pretty much on our own. We simply don't know how to deal with our emotions, either when they're actually arising or in their aftermaths. Nor do we grasp the immense harm done, both to ourselves and to everyone around us, by this lack of understanding.

To be fair, the situation has begun to improve. During the nineties, the term "emotional intelligence" took hold. This term is usually defined as the ability to monitor, regulate, and obtain information from our feelings. It was popularized in a landmark book of the same name by *New York Times* writer Daniel Goleman. Since then, emotions have been dragged out of the closet and into the open at progressive schools, institutions, and businesses worldwide. Where it once was taboo, the topic is now generally recognized as a key to effective communication, organization, and even a robust bottom line.

This is a great beginning, and the benefits of emotional intelligence will only continue to spread. But emotional intelligence is just half of what's necessary. The other half, perhaps even more important, is emotional connection.

Emotional connection is the ability not just to recognize an emotion, but to actually feel it. And not just to feel it for a moment, or for as long as it's comfortable, but for as long as that specific emotion requires.

This practice is simple and direct. It can be learned and mastered in a short time by almost anyone. It's the key to maximizing all talent and effort. It's the key to making dreams come true. And yet, emotional connection remains the road *least* traveled.

Why? Both nature and nurture, as previously alluded to, play large roles. But the complete answer goes further than that. To let our emotions run their own course, in their own time, necessitates a radical shift of consciousness. We must overcome a pervasive view that emotions are best kept in check, that they are the enemies of rational thinking, and that to give them fuller reign would lead to anarchy, weakness, or the kind of touchy-feely navel gazing that makes even the most tolerant among us wince.

Do you believe that too? Perhaps just a little? Most of us do, even if we don't like to admit it, and even if we've learned to give lip service to "feeling our feelings" at Twelve Step programs, in counseling, or somewhere else along the way.

In this book, I challenge the view that emotions are problems, that they're things to be feared, controlled, or even managed by our "higher" faculties. I make the case, instead, that emotional connection is the path to our greatest possible wisdom and achievement, no matter what the field of endeavor. I do so, mostly, by appealing to your own common sense and experience.

The first time I shared this approach was in an article for the September 2004 issue of *O, The Oprah Magazine*. In response, e-mails poured in from all over the world. The general consensus went something like this: "Everything you're saying is obvious. Yet somehow I'd missed it. More, please."

It's in response to those requests that I set out to write *The One Thing Holding You Back.* My goal is to provide all the principles and practices you need in order to make emotional connection a regular part of your life. I want to help you put emotional connection to use, not just in general, but also wherever you may be stuck, and to empower any and all of your dreams. In fact, the central message of the book is this:

> To whatever degree you aren't living your dreams, it's because of key emotions related to those dreams that you're not yet able to find and feel. Once you're able, those dreams will begin to come true in one form or another.

This is, no doubt, a bold claim. And I make it in a way that's even bolder than you might think. I'm not just referring to personal accomplishment but to the objectives of groups and companies as well. Here are two brief examples that illustrate how emotional connection can become the critical missing link in reaching personal and collective goals.

First, imagine a lonely woman who wants nothing more than a loving relationship but has become gun-shy due to previous rejection. While caution in relationships is always a good thing, in her case it's blown up into a paralyzing fear. This unwillingness to feel any possible rejection causes her to bail out on new partners before things ever have a chance to get serious. Therefore, she unwittingly ensures her isolation.

Next, take the case of a manager and his team, working within a large company. They're behind in their sales targets, and the manager's job is on the line. He's unwilling to experience even the slightest tinge of failure, however, so when presented with important information about serious obstacles facing his team, he throws a temper tantrum. The team members, for their part, are unwilling to experience the humiliation that results from these tantrums. Gradually, they hide more and more bad news from the manager until their paltry earnings report comes out and the whole department is downsized.

These examples illustrate the consequences of saying no to an emotional experience. And they lead us to another essential message of this book:

Whenever you're not willing to experience a particular emotion, your life is run by your resistance to that emotion. You make choices that are about avoiding the feeling, rather than serving your best interests. Emotional resistance, therefore, is the one thing holding you back.

Emotions make the world go round. They're at the root of all our dreams. Resistance to emotions brings those dreams to a screeching halt. This uneasy dance between emotions and emotional resistance is always present, usually behind the scenes, enormously influential as the drama of life plays out.

But what about saying yes to emotions? How do things change for the better when we release our resistance and experience greater emotional connection? For a first-pass answer to this question, let's revisit our examples.

In the case of the lonely woman, her willingness to feel rejection would increase the odds that she could sustain a relationship. Beyond that basic goal, she'd also be able to see prospective partners through a wider, less rejection-focused lens. This, in turn, would help improve the ultimate suitability of the men she chose to pursue.

Regarding the corporate manager and his sales force, a willingness to experience failure and humiliation would give them the opportunity to clear the air and create an environment of greater trust and collaboration. In addition, they'd be better able to identify and shore up any actual team weaknesses.

Throughout this book, I'll continually amplify the benefits of emotional connection. I'll also provide many real examples, from all walks of life, in which people have practiced emotional connection and seen profound results. Whether you're trying to lose weight, make millions, end world hunger, or communicate with your teenager, you'll find applicable stories in these pages. Their inspiration and the tools they demonstrate will help bring your own goals to fruition.

I do, however, need to make one vital clarification. The claim I've made about emotional connection is that it will make your dreams come true *in one form or another*. This doesn't mean that if you dream about earning millions and practice emotional connection, you'll go on to rake in all that cash. You might, but that's not really the point. The point—and the promise—is that you'll experience a major shift. You'll free up your creative energy, distill your vision, improve your follow-through, and work much, much smarter. Along the way, as a result, you'll come to feel like a million bucks no matter what happens.

Likewise, if you're aiming to get rid of serious chronic pain, I can't guarantee that employing emotional connection will make that happen. But what I can assure you is that even if it doesn't, you'll be able to handle your pain with greater ease and quality of life.

The reason I'm able to make such confident assertions is that emotional connection is what I teach in my workshops. I do it around the world, with all kinds of people. I've held workshops at the poshest spas and at the starkest prisons. In every situation, I witness the same outcome—the simple, straightforward act of feeling creates lasting and remarkable breakthroughs. This happens even when people have tried everything else previously, when they've given up all hope of real change. That's because emotional connection isn't yet another technique. Nor does it supply something you're missing. Instead, emotional connection is a doorway to your own innate, untapped potential. In other words, it will bring forth and support the very best of what's already in you.

As you read on to discover how this works, I encourage you not to take anything I say on faith. Be rigorous. Test out what you find here in the laboratory of your own life. The finest outcome, from my perspective, is that you alter these principles and practices in whatever ways fit you best.

We'll begin with a warm-up and a definition of terms. I'll ask you to do a few simple experiments that ground those definitions in your own experience. Then, in part 2, I'll provide you with the tools and information necessary to begin exercising your muscle of emotional connection. In part 3, as that muscle strengthens, you'll learn to apply it directly to the areas of your life where it's time for moving mountains. I'll walk you carefully through every step of that process, providing special tips for those moments and situations where a breakthrough may seem virtually impossible.

Part 4 includes detailed profiles of people putting emotional connection to work for their own breakthroughs. Chapter 10 focuses on overcoming addictions and compulsions such as smoking and overeating. Chapter 11 covers a wide variety of work-related issues such as a difficult boss, unfulfilling career path, and outsourcing. Chapter 12 deals with relationship and communication, examining three generations of a family in crisis.

Some of these profiles may seem more relevant to your situation than others, but I encourage you to read them all carefully. That's because each profile contains at least one "key refinement" to the emotional-connection process. No matter what specific challenges you face, these key refinements will help boost your success. They'll get you through the inevitable messy parts, when it's all too easy to fall back on previous conditioning.

Chapter 13 imagines a future in which all of us, and especially our political leaders, put emotional connection to use with transformative results. Appendix A addresses the remaining concerns that participants ask about most often in workshops and individual sessions. Appendix B, for easy reference, provides a brief rundown of all the practices and refinements presented throughout the book.

By the time you finish this book, there will be *nothing* holding you back. You'll recognize your emotions quickly, feel them fully, and take their wisdom to heart. Your internal resources will be strengthened and harmonized for peak impact. As a result, you'll meet life's inevitable challenges with ease, flexibility, and a joyful, creative spirit. Rather than just reaching your goals, you'll exceed them.

That's the power of emotional connection. Now, let's put it to work for you.

PART ONE

GETTING
READY

~ I ~

WHAT IS AN EMOTION, ANYWAY?

S INCE OUR JOURNEY BEGINS and ends with emotional connection, it would help to have a clear working definition of what an
emotion actually is. But that's a problem, because neither philosophers
nor psychologists nor scientists can come to agreement. They contest
one another's definitions vigorously across disciplines and even more
so within them. So where does that leave us?

Fortunately, we don't really need to enter the fray. That's because
emotions are are much easier to experience than describe. It's usually
not too difficult to know that you're angry, for example, even if you're
uncertain about the neurological and biochemical processes that produce such anger. For our purposes, the ever-evolving theories and
squabbles about how to define emotion are only relevant to the extent
that they bolster the ability, and the commitment, to feel. In that regard,
there are a few important topics to consider.

The first is the purpose of emotion. All schools of thought agree that
emotions exist to convey information. Emotions arise as a response to the

changing states of our internal and external environments. They're part of the overall process that helps us understand our world and ourselves.

PURPOSE OF EMOTION

External Change $\longrightarrow$ Emotion Conveys Response
(e.g., an insult)   *(e.g., hurt)*

Internal Change $\longrightarrow$ Emotion Conveys Response
(e.g., missing a friend)   *(e.g., sadness)*

FIGURE 1

Just now, I took a break from writing to do the dishes. Midway through, I broke a crystal champagne flute that was given to me by a past partner. At first I seemed to take it in stride. These things happen, I thought. No big deal. But when I tuned in to my emotions, I suddenly felt flushed and sad. Retrieving a broom and dustpan, I replayed the tumultuous ending of that relationship. My heart beat faster. Tears welled. I realized, with surprise, that I wasn't totally healed from the breakup. My emotional response, in this case, enabled me to refine my self-understanding.

Along with their role in understanding, emotions also serve to inform and influence our needs, drives, perceptions, and perhaps most of all, actions. The word "emotion" itself is formed from the Latin roots *ex* and *motio,* signifying outward movement. This underscores the way that emotions form a vital bridge between self-identity and self-expression. In other words, they help us glean both who we are and how best to conduct our lives.

That is, of course, when everything's working properly. Another thing widely agreed upon by scholars is that emotions are not always reliable. They're part instinctive and part learned. If a person grew up in a war zone, for example, the sound of a sonic boom in later life might produce an excessive amount of fear. Or, conversely, a person who grew up in a gated community might not feel afraid *enough* in a bad neighborhood. In both cases early emotional development could lead to an incorrect interpretation of later circumstances.

On the other hand, who's to say what's a "correct" emotional response to anything? What to one person feels like a small mishap might feel downright tragic to another. The range and intensity of emotions we experience are influenced not just by the past but also by culture, personality, and even physiology. Therefore, emotions aren't ever entirely right or wrong, good or bad, reliable or fallible.

CORE CONCEPT

Emotions aren't ever entirely right or wrong, good or bad, reliable or fallible.

Instead, their initial arising presents raw, unprocessed feedback. Most emotions take shape for all of us in this same self-generating way, whether or not we want their input or approve of their message.

What happens next, once an emotion has arisen, is really the crux of the matter. At this stage we have an array of choices. We can talk about it, act it out unconsciously, or deny it completely. We can suppress it, interpret it, debate it, or obsess about it. Or, more simply, we can just allow ourselves to stay aware of it.

Soon we'll examine all of these choices as well as many more. For now, let's focus on the last one. To stay aware of an emotion that has arisen within us is sometimes not as easy as it sounds, since many of us are adept at blocking out feelings we don't want. And yet emotions are constantly forming within us whether we're aware of them fully, briefly, or not at all. When we're unaware, we rob ourselves of whatever information emotions have to impart. Therefore, the conventional preference for rationality over emotion makes no sense. For the greatest degree of success in tackling life's challenges and realizing our dreams, we need both.

My client Vivian illustrates this well. She told me she was "born to sing." Ever since high school her secret wish was to put together a nightclub act. But the years drifted by, and three kids came along, each one offering a convenient new excuse to put her singing on the back burner.

Looking at the situation rationally, Vivian had always seen her problem as standard-issue procrastination. This theory, however, never helped her get moving.

In our work together, while reflecting on her long-stalled dream, Vivian experienced waves of anger and disappointment. At first she thought these feelings were about not following through with her dream, but soon the real answer dawned—her voice was mediocre. Despite her passion for singing, Vivian possessed no remarkable talent.

Until accessing all the emotions that preceded this truth, Vivian was never able to find or face it. Even the clearest, soberest thinking had been no match for her giant blind spot. Now, accepting her mediocrity rather than resisting it, she was actually relieved. Unburdened of false diva-hood, she could thoroughly reassess her voice for all its true strengths and weaknesses. She did this with the aid of a voice coach, who also helped her select a repertoire that highlighted her strengths. Within six months Vivian was singing at open mikes, and within another six months she performed her first full set.

CORE CONCEPT

**Emotions contain information that
thoughts alone can't.**

To accurately discern our emotions, as Vivian did, we need to know where they appear. The answer is obvious but has been downplayed and even ignored for centuries. Emotions are physical. They arise and fade away in our bodies. That's the one and only place emotions can ever be found.

When the dominant Western religions deemed the body a source of evil, they also cast suspicion on emotion. Five of the seven deadly sins—pride, envy, lust, anger, and greed—actually *are* emotions. Likewise, when the rise of science fostered an inordinate emphasis on logic and a belief that the body existed merely to support the brain, emotions took another blow. While the advent of holistic health and emotional intelligence has done much to redress this, for the vast majority the body still remains a foreign and seemingly chaotic place. As a result, even if we choose to, most of us don't really know *how* to feel.

CORE CONCEPT

Emotions are physical. Our bodies are the only place they can ever be found.

Without knowing how to feel, it's impossible to determine what we truly want, why we want it, and how to successfully pursue it. Whether at home, work, or play, we simply can't be our best. With that knowledge, on the other hand, everything becomes clearer and easier. That's why emotional connection—and the specific skills you'll learn in this book— is even more powerful than it first appears.

Emotions are like weather, constantly passing through the landscape of your physical body. To experience the subtle changes in that weather, you need to develop a close and attentive relationship with your body. Especially, you need to develop a keen awareness of your internal physical sensations.

In fact, there is no immediate and foolproof way to distinguish between an internal sensation that's emotionally related and one that isn't. Think about it—that gnawing in your stomach may be a gut feeling, or just as possibly indigestion. Only time and sustained attention can render a clear distinction. Learning to make such distinctions is what allows you to maximize your personal feedback system. That's why our investigation of the one thing holding you back will be primarily body centered.

Another reason for focusing on the body is that most of us have been deeply conditioned to believe we control it. Whether for purposes of health, vanity, or both, we invest extravagant amounts of time and money to get results from our bodies, to bend them to our wills. In the process we forget all about things like converting food to energy and purifying blood, things that bodies do *for* us on their own and that we could never perform by choice. As a result, we tend to ignore our bodies when we don't perceive a problem and then fixate upon them when we do.

To foster and maintain emotional connection requires that we become curious, rather than suspicious, about our bodies. When experiencing an unpleasant internal sensation, we must exchange the usual knee-jerk approach—"What's wrong?! How do I get rid of it?!"—for one of humility and respect. We need to experience our bodies' messages as complex, subtle, and, above all, *worthy* of sustained attention. Only then, with the body as ally instead of servant, will emotional connection bear fruit.

This doesn't mean, as we'll soon see, that your job is to decode your body's messages. For example, if sustained attention to the pain in your chest reveals it as heartbreak, not heartburn, you don't then have to figure that heartbreak out. The act of figuring out is mental and actually serves to remove you from your emotions. Your only job, throughout this book, will be to keep noticing what you feel. Noticing will lead you to realize that emotions *are* the messages. To notice an emotion fully is to experience it fully. At that point the message is received, and no further work is necessary.

PRACTICAL TIP

> **Your only job, throughout this book, will be to keep noticing what you feel. To notice an emotion fully is to experience it fully. At that point the message is received, and no further work is necessary.**

Any additional meaning you garner from emotional connection will come naturally, with no effort whatsoever, as a gift for relating to yourself in this way. That's exactly what happened to me regarding the champagne flute and to Vivian regarding her voice.

Throughout the book, when describing how to notice your sensations, I'll use the terms "feelings" and "emotions" interchangeably. Some experts keep the two separate, using "feeling" to refer to sensory experience only and "emotion" to include both sensory experience and our subsequent evaluation of it. In other words, their idea is that a complete emotion is comprised of a feeling itself and then also all our thoughts about that feeling. But it's my contention that we can only think the most clearly and successfully about an emotion after we sense it, and after sensing it for much longer than most of us are accustomed. By perhaps over-emphasizing the sensory component of our emotional experiences, I hope to bring the whole picture into better balance.

MINDING YOUR BODY

We've been discussing sensations and emotions for a while, so let's turn now to your own experience of these phenomena. It's best to read the following instructions all the way through before actually beginning the practice.

Place your attention on your body. Notice if any sensation stands out. Do you feel something particular in your belly, chest, limbs, or head? Let whatever your attention lands on first be the focus for this exercise. Keep your attention on that sensation for a few moments, watching closely to see how it changes. Avoid the temptation to name it or to influence it in any way.

Does it move or stay fixed? Does it change a little or a lot? Does it lessen or intensify? Or, perhaps, does it seem to remain exactly the same?

See if you can stay in this gentle, inquisitive, nondefining mode for at least a minute. If your attention wanders or mind chatter begins to take over, just acknowledge what's happening and return to your sensation once again.

At the end of the minute, consider whether the sensation has an emotional quality to it. If it does, and you know what the emotion is, note that. If you don't know what the emotion is, note that too. If the sensation doesn't seem to have an emotional quality, or you can't tell for sure, just let it remain without any further analysis or description.

No matter what you experience—stay relaxed. There is absolutely no way to do any of this exploration wrong. You're simply exercising

*your bodily awareness and remaining attentive to what your aware-
ness locates. The "muscle" at work is the exact one necessary for emotional connection.*

*If you turn your attention to your body and notice no sensation
whatsoever, still stay relaxed. There's no error or problem. It just
means that at this moment nothing is strong enough to call your attention or that perhaps you're a little numb. In either case, just keep gently
scanning your body from head to toe until something shows up. It may
be as simple as an itch on the knee, or the rise and fall of your breath.
Whatever draws your attention eventually (and something always
will), stay with that as you continue the exercise.*

*Before moving on, take a moment to assess the current state of your
body-awareness muscle. Based on the exercise, is it weak or strong?
Foreign or familiar? Are you primed to learn more about it and to
work it systematically? Or does the whole arena seem daunting? Let
your honest answers to these questions guide you in how quickly to
keep going through the rest of the book. If you feel at all like a fish out
of water, go slowly. Though it may not make sense just yet, that's the
fastest way to get results.*

In this first chapter, we've seen that emotions play an instrumental
role in how we relate to ourselves and the world. Emotions usually arise
of their own accord. While not always true indicators of what's happening or how best to respond, they are essential in reaching the greatest
possible understanding of who we are and what we want. Located in
the body, emotions make themselves known primarily through internal
sensations. The more attuned we grow to these internal sensations, the
wiser and more discriminating we become.

But the benefits of emotional connection are far greater than that.
Whenever we've grown stale, emotions reawaken us. Wherever we've
become stuck, they get us moving. With just the simple ability to notice
and experience our feelings—which you're about to master in complete, practical detail—daily existence becomes fascinating and vibrant.
We shift from lethargic to motivated, from passive to energized. Life
becomes a grand adventure of which we're author and hero both.

~ 2 ~

YEAH, BUT

I F YOU'VE READ THIS FAR, most likely there's at least a part of you that's interested in learning more about emotional connection. But there also may be a part of you that's not so sure. This ambivalence is normal and widespread. It's actually healthy, in that our instinctive brains (as we'll cover later) try to protect us from any experiences they consider dangerous. The defense mechanisms our instinctive brains employ in this effort are quite sophisticated and usually unconscious.

I experienced this personally during my early twenties. By all accounts I was emotion friendly. When struggling with their feelings, people often sought me out for the nonjudgmental support I was eager to provide. They'd want to know how I came to be so emotionally adept and stable and how I'd "escaped" from the harmful legacy of my childhood. Proudly, I responded to their inquiries with a recitation of the coping strategies I devised along the way. In truth, while these strategies were real, they did nothing at all to prevent the hurt of my upbringing. Years later, after a series of failed relationships led me to therapy, I discovered the serious emotional wounding that had been present all along.

By their very nature, unconscious defenses aren't yet available to our awareness. But there's a reliable indicator if they're afoot within you—any type of explanation about why emotional connection isn't relevant or appropriate for your own unrealized goals. Such an explanation, or a "Yeah, but" as I call it, can undermine your efforts at emotional connection before they even get started. So in the spirit of gently disarming whatever defenses you may possess, let's tackle some of the most prevalent "yeah, buts" head-on.

1. Yeah, but I'm a man. We're just not made for the whole emotions thing.

There's at least a little truth in this. Most men, due both to gender and socialization, have a difficult time with vulnerability. And vulnerability is absolutely necessary in order to feel emotions fully. In addition, men tend to be more removed than women from their overall bodily experiences. After all, men don't menstruate or bear children and can therefore get away with a little distance. Finally, even when they do connect with bodily sensations, men more typically find a range and degree of feeling less pronounced than their female counterparts.

However, all that just means that men have more of a challenge in this arena, not that they're incapable. Take Gary, for instance. He's a cop, and when I met him, he wanted more than anything not to lose Jennifer, his wife of twenty-six years. But she was fed up with his gruff, impassive, stone-cold approach to life. Things had reached a peak when their teenage son was expelled from school. Jennifer was devastated and couldn't understand why Gary didn't care. Gary bought in to this view of himself, too, since all the stuff he was supposed to feel and express seemed like totally foreign territory.

I suggested that Gary put aside, just for a moment, the idea that he was somehow deficient. I asked him to tell me exactly how his son got expelled. I pressed him for details and then directed him to scan his body for any sensation whatsoever. Gary told me that his shoulders were tense, his neck was throbbing, and his cheeks felt prickly and hot.

"That's it!" I proclaimed. "Tell Jennifer that." Gary looked at me quizzically. I explained that these simple physical sensations were just the type of emotional response they'd both given up on. A glimmer of hope crossed his face. He did tell Jennifer. It was a start. From there, Gary quickly learned how to reveal more. A few years later he and Jennifer are still together. He continues to freeze and clam up from time to time, but since Jennifer can clearly see his commitment, she's usually willing to cut him some slack.

If you're a man, rest assured that emotional connection will not require you to shed one iota of your masculinity or power. Instead, it will put you more in touch with yourself, clarify the path to your goals, and liberate your potential to achieve them.

2. Yeah, but I'm a woman, and I already know this stuff. If anything, I feel too much.

This one's partially true as well. Women *are* natural-born feelers. But what they often do with feelings can be just as damaging as what men do. After touching the raw sensation of an emotion ever so briefly, they may try to escape by talking about it with friends, writing about it in a journal, or "processing" it in therapy. They may get lost in analyzing, interpreting, rationalizing, or defending against the feeling. In addition they may distract themselves with a dramatic reaction to it. Finally, they may get caught up in judgment and blame, either of the person who triggered the emotion or of themselves for having it.

To be fair, some of the above responses to emotion can actually be very helpful. But if they're called upon to get rid of a feeling, rather than embrace it, any possible benefit is thwarted. The point here is that being emotionally oriented, as so many women are, is not at all the same as being emotionally connected. That distinction, if not entirely clear, will take center stage in part 2.

Another common female response to an emotion is the opposite— clinging to it much longer than necessary. In other words, the emotion itself is ready to release before the person experiencing it will let that happen. I came across a classic case of this scenario with Haruko, who compared her situation to trading in an old car for a new one. She said, in this regard, that she was "upside down." I wasn't familiar with this term and asked her to explain it.

"If you owe more on your current car than it's worth," she said, "the dealer calls that being upside down. Well, that's how I am with my past relationship. It only lasted for a year, but I've been grieving it for two. And I know it's getting in the way of finding my true life partner."

After a brief exploration, it became clear to Haruko that she'd held on to the grief so long because it was the last thing connecting her to this man. With that understanding and about a minute of tears, she felt the grief dissipate and was now totally ready to move on. Nothing more was required. Just two minutes of emotional connection accomplished what two years of clinging never could.

3. Yeah, but if my emotions are such a problem, why shouldn't I just take medication?

Each year in this country millions upon millions of prescriptions are dispensed for antidepressant and antianxiety medication. For some these medications are true lifesavers. For others they provide temporary buffers in times of great pain. But for many they're misapplied and ineffective, leaving people with serious side effects and the unfortunate impression that they're *beyond* help.

For me, depression and anxiety aren't emotional conditions, but rather responses to emotional upset. Depression is usually just what it sounds like—a pushing down of feeling. The resulting listlessness comes from having to expend so much energy in an effort to keep difficult emotions from surfacing. The best description I know for anxiety, in a similar vein, is the fear *of* feeling. Creating a pervasive state of agitation is a way, conscious or not, to avoid the uncomfortable emotion that underlies it.

The prevalent medical view is that if depression or anxiety persists for a significant period of time, then the situation is clinical and drugs are appropriate. But if there isn't any real effort made to break through these states with direct emotional connection, then it's impossible to know whether their continuation is due to true mental illness or merely entrenched resistance.

Since I'm not a physician, I don't dispense medical advice or seek to influence my clients' decisions regarding medication. But I do have one suggestion that usually helps people make those decisions with greater clarity and confidence: when facing significant depression or anxiety, learn the practice of emotional connection, and apply it consistently for at least a couple of weeks. If your distress continues regardless, then it's definitely time to see the doctor.

But most frequently that's not what happens. Instead, emotional connection liberates all the energy and well-being previously sapped by depression or anxiety. People feel revitalized, peaceful, and well equipped to handle difficult emotions the next time they arise. Plus, they're relieved not to have been clinically ill after all. And for those who eventually do receive a diagnosis, the ability to connect emotionally still improves their handling of life's inevitable stressful passages. It also helps wean them off medication, when appropriate, with greater ease and speed.

When Connie came to see me, she was already on an antidepressant. "All the energy had just drained out of my life," she told me. "I used to be a happy, productive person, but now there's just no spark." During the appointment, our conversation kept coming back to Josh, her disabled fourteen-year-old son. Josh was adorable but also out of control and infuriating. For years, Connie resisted huge amounts of anger toward him because it "wasn't right" to be angry at someone who "couldn't help it." I guided Connie to separate her judgment about this anger from the raw fact of its existence. I suggested that her depression was a natural result of keeping the lid on so much rage.

To remedy the situation, I suggested that Connie carry around a notepad and make a tally mark every time Josh's behavior elicited a new surge of anger. Each tally mark represented five minutes of any anger-expression technique—her choice—to be performed as soon as Connie could arrange for alone time. She usually opted for dancing and hollering to aggressive music. Some days required only ten minutes of such discharge, but others up to an hour. Soon, Connie had learned to release her anger quickly, close to its arising, and had also emptied herself of a decade-long backlog. As a result, her verve returned. She and her doctor decided to discontinue medication. The following autumn Connie went back to school to complete a long-delayed degree program in special education.

4. Yeah, but the work I do requires me to suppress emotion. To feel it would actually sabotage my goals.

There are, indeed, times and places that are entirely inappropriate for emotional connection. No one wants a surgeon who pauses, mid-procedure, to mourn the loss of his pet. But the important thing to recall here—and we'll take a closer look at it soon—is that our emotions arise whether we're aware of them or not. They don't clear out of our physiological and psychological systems unless we give them the opportunity to do so. Whenever our personal or group responsibilities require that we temporarily stave off emotion, "Not now, later" is a fitting and effective approach. Unfortunately, most of us go on to forget the "later" part. As the following example illustrates, over time this can do great damage to our on-the-job performance.

Gloria is a lawyer in the district attorney's office of a prominent Southern city. Her greatest ambition is to *be* the district attorney. A couple of years ago she came to a workshop, wary and defiant. "My job demands that I deny my emotions all day long—so whaddaya got for me?" I smiled understandingly and suggested she stick around, take nothing on faith, and just keep an open mind. Grudgingly, she consented.

That night, after she felt much safer, Gloria decided to share a disturbing story. She recalled having to put a six-year-old girl on the witness stand before a grand jury, in order to acquire a sexual-abuse indictment against the girl's father. It felt, to Gloria, that her detailed line of questioning had forced the girl to relive the horrific experience. Relaying this, hard-as-nails Gloria suddenly began to sob uncontrollably. A few minutes later, when her tears and guilt subsided, she looked up and whispered to the group. "This happened a year and a half ago, and till now I hadn't said a word about it to anybody."

Once she grew calm, I suggested to Gloria that keeping such emotion locked up is a surefire recipe for burnout. She nodded, admitting to a few recent uncharacteristic courtroom defeats. How frequently she put the "Not now, later" formula to use was up to her, I explained, but at least some regular schedule—nightly, weekly, monthly—was imperative.

And in my experience there's neither an individual nor a profession for which the same suggestion isn't equally effective.

5. Yeah, but I take control of my emotions.
I don't let them take control of me.

This mind-over-emotion approach usually takes one of three forms. The first is popular in what's loosely termed the New Age community, where it's presumed that we create our ongoing reality with the power and intention of our thoughts. Placing one's focus on difficult or negative emotions, from this perspective, seems like a way to perpetuate suffering rather than alleviate it.

In my extensive work with people who share this orientation, I've found a significant confusion between fixating on emotions and accepting them. The former, in fact, always does perpetuate suffering, while the latter creates the environment of inner harmony best suited to successful positive thinking. In other words, emotional connection aids, rather than impedes, a mind-centered approach.

Ursula, for instance, had one clear goal—to reach the top of the corporate ladder at the multinational energy company where she'd worked for twelve years. Every day Ursula spoke affirmations and performed visualizations to imagine herself in an executive suite. When we met, however, she was stuck in middle management and saddled with a reputation as a "glory hog" who habitually overemphasized her own contributions, minimized those of coworkers, and often took illegitimate credit for the success of others. Three times, when Ursula had been passed over for VP, her selfish reputation was cited as a main cause. Privately, with a sense of confusion and regret, Ursula admitted to me that it was all true. She felt as if there was a "monster" that kept hijacking her brain. It made her cutthroat, irrational, and greedy for every scrap of praise.

In the service of a breakthrough, I asked Ursula not to fight the monster, but instead to give it temporary free reign within her until she could sense its purpose. She paused a long time, then reported, "It needs a role to play, something to contribute." And if none of that were possible, I wondered, how would Ursula feel? She took another moment and then replied, "Absolutely unlovable."

Resisting this unlovable feeling was the one thing holding Ursula back from achieving her goal. The emotion itself came from a brutal childhood that included drug-addicted parents and abusive foster caregivers. It took a lot of motivation and courage for Ursula to let herself finally feel it. Once she did, however, the emotion began to subside after just a couple of sessions. In the months following, Ursula came to see that lovability was innate, not something that any of us has to earn. At that point it became easy to let her colleagues bask in their full share of the limelight. Meanwhile, her affirmations and visualizations took on a more vibrant, magnetic quality. A year later, when the next VP position opened up, Ursula was the consensus first choice.

The second mind-over-emotion version comes from the world of cognitive psychology, where it's often theorized that unpleasant feelings are produced by incorrect beliefs and that by changing those beliefs, we can eliminate the feelings at their source. This does work sometimes, and investigating our beliefs is always a helpful pursuit. In particular, when our emotional response to a situation is out of date or otherwise miscalibrated, we definitely need a broader perspective to set things right. Ursula, clearly, possessed an old, unexamined belief that personal worth depends upon the validation of others. We spoke about this belief frequently, and updating it with a healthier one was definitely part of our plan.

Yet, what gave rise to that belief in the first place was that Ursula truly *felt* unlovable. The emotion itself was her evidence. Had she attempted to update her belief without first experiencing and releasing that emotion, it wouldn't have been more than a band-aid measure. At the first serious setback, despite all her mental effort, this new belief would simply have dissolved into the same old emotional soup. What Ursula's example demonstrates, especially regarding our most intractable negative beliefs, is that they're often a by-product of our unresolved emotions. In these cases it's the emotions that produce the beliefs, not the other way around. Cognitive psychology, therefore, tends to be the most successful when preceded and accompanied by sufficient emotional connection.

The third mind-over-emotion version is religious and counsels that we employ the power of petitionary prayer to ask God for help in relieving our distress. I've had many people waver on attending an emotional-connection workshop because they're worried that it's anti-God or that so much self-empowerment heretically conveys a godlike stature on human beings.

My response is that emotional connection is the best way I know to open the heart and therefore to help us all hear and heed the message of whatever God we worship. No one I've encountered who learned and mastered the tools of emotional connection ever went on to reject them on religious grounds. To the contrary, many religious people have found emotional connection indispensable in deepening their faith.

6. Yeah, but all this is nothing new. It's called meditation.

Most of the world's meditation traditions have lots to teach about acceptance of whatever arises in the present moment. Buddhism, in particular, is based largely on this practice. But when it comes to emotion, things get a little murky. Most schools of meditation, while strong on emotional awareness, also caution seriously against emotional excess. They offer techniques to develop inner peace and a capacity to witness emotions rather than being swept up by them.

PRACTICAL TIP

Emotional connection requires both complete immersion and complete awareness.

No problem there, except that emotions, in particular, need more than witnessing. They need to be felt. They need complete immersion and complete awareness equally, simultaneously. Otherwise meditation can render us passive and remote, which in turn diminishes, rather than enhances, our will to succeed.

So to those of you with a lot of meditation experience and a "been there, done that" perspective, I suggest considering this book's approach a subtle but fundamental course correction. Skim what feels familiar, and focus on what's different. Allow yourself the chance to take an up-to-date emotional assessment, paying special attention to those feelings you habitually resist. Releasing your greatest resistance, always, uncovers your greatest treasure.

Even if you're now clear about the necessity of emotional connection and your "yeah, buts" have been sufficiently resolved, you may still remain wary about the whole realm of emotions. This wariness is completely understandable. Remember how earlier I suggested that emotions are similar to weather? That's true in an additional way I haven't yet discussed. Emotions, like weather, are totally unpredictable. In just a split second, your peaceful internal climate can become blustery and torrential. No wonder we so often seek refuge within the less charged shelter of our thoughts. From within that shelter it can seem that we're in the best position to address our wants and needs—even emotional ones—with the aid of restraint and distance.

If you're entirely satisfied with this approach and the results it's produced, then there's really no reason to read on. But if you sense that you're capable of more and that life is also, then I invite you to consider a middle path between distance and deluge. When carefully attended to, the great force of the elements—sun, wind, and rain—bestows upon us the energy to transform our world. So, too, with emotions. In the next section you'll learn precisely how to channel emotional energy into personal achievement and maximum well-being. You'll discover how to safely and successfully navigate through even the most daunting emotional storms. Instead of avoiding such storms, you'll actually begin to seek them out. Right there, amid the very downpour, you'll soak up all the nutrients to grow.

PART TWO

FEELING AND NOT FEELING

3

HOW TO FEEL

EMOTIONAL CONNECTION is a natural phenomenon. As human beings, we're wired for it. When you read about it in this chapter, your response may be something like, "Of course. That makes total sense." Yet the topic also requires specific instruction. That's because emotional resistance, which is just as natural, causes us to forget all about the fundamentals of feeling.

In describing exactly how to feel, I've developed a model that's simple to remember and apply. This model was tested and refined over eight years during private sessions and public workshops with thousands of individuals from all walks of life. It's called the 2 X 2 process. The first 2 explains what to do, and the second 2 explains how to do it. With the what and how together, emotional connection is entirely effective in most situations. Apart from each other, neither can stand completely on its own. Once you've read through the explanation below, consult the 2 X 2 process diagram on page 35 for easy reference. Now, keeping all that in mind, let's dive in.

Step 1   To experience an emotion, place your attention directly on the sensation it produces in your body.

Step 2   Keep your attention on that sensation until it either dissipates or changes.

That's all there is to the first "2." Really. These two simple steps, however, are often anything but easy. To perform them well, especially at the most difficult times, requires two corresponding shifts in the quality of our attention. These shifts, described below, comprise the second part of the 2 X 2 process.

Shift One: Slow Down

Our instant-gratification culture has drastically shortened the average human attention span. When most of us turn our attention to physical and emotional sensations, we have a simultaneous expectation that all will be divulged quickly. When it isn't, we tend to lose interest, give up, or get down on ourselves. But emotions are prone to reveal themselves slowly, like an unraveling ball of yarn.

Cecilia was a commercial real-estate broker. She had an appointment to see a customer with a big sale on the line. The appointment had been on her calendar for over a month, yet she'd procrastinated the whole time and done none of the necessary preparation. Cecilia called me in a panic a few hours before the appointment, just as unprepared and yet still unable to apply herself. She needed to know, with so much at stake, how to break through her untimely paralysis. I suggested that she tune in to her emotions for insight. Performing Step 1, she noticed a fluttery sensation in her stomach.

"I'm nervous," she deduced but was thoroughly unimpressed. "Didn't need the jitters to tell me that." Her usual MO in such circumstances would be to tune back out and continue fumbling her way toward the appointment. Instead, I suggested she pause long enough to perform Step 2. What she experienced went something like this:

> The fluttery feeling is starting to bubble up to my chest. My heart's beating quickly too. Okay, now all that's subsiding, and there's a sinking sensation in my diaphragm. It makes me want to curl into a ball. Whoa, this feeling is really familiar. It's the same thing that

happens every time I have to visit my father-in-law. Come to think of it, this guy totally reminds me of my father-in-law . . . the way he's so dismissive and demeaning.

With the "ball of yarn" unraveled, Cecilia now saw through her nervousness to the source of it. With this information it became much easier to separate the past from the present and the personal from the professional. Only by setting aside her need for a quick fix was Cecilia then able to efficiently address the business at hand. But truthfully, even a scenario like this one doesn't typically take more than a minute or two. With a little practice, therefore, the required slowdown isn't even all that slow.

To make this depiction of a slowdown complete, we need to shade in one particular detail. The important insight about Cecilia's father-in-law was a thought, not a feeling, but that thought arose *through* the process of feeling. Had Cecilia started to think about the situation without feeling, or at any time before the nervousness evolved into a sinking sensation, it's unlikely that the same conclusion would have dawned.

Most of us make the mistake of trying to figure out a situation just mentally, and too soon, before all the insights that emotions lead to can make themselves known. So the slowdown isn't only necessary for emotions to run their course, but also to create the greatest possible synergy between feeling and thinking.

Thinking is our most extraordinary tool, but only at the right place and time. In fact, trying to figure out a feeling too soon is usually an attempt to get rid of it.

CORE CONCEPT

Trying to figure out a feeling too soon is often an effort to get rid of it.

And whenever we pit thoughts and feelings against each other in such a fashion, we upset their delicate balance. This only serves to make us less aware, not more, and therefore defeats our initial purpose entirely.

Shift Two: Get Microscopic

In describing this shift, I always find it best to begin with ants. It really perks up drifting seminar participants to ask them how human beings ever came to know the detailed workings of an anthill. The answer, in large part, is that hundreds of scientists parked themselves next to anthills and just watched. And watched and watched. They peered through a magnifying glass, searching for every observable detail. Over time, what began looking like a blob of indistinguishable activity eventually came into focus. Without doing anything to change the behavior of the ants, the scientists were able to perceive new and vital details. Long after the process seemed complete, long after it seemed there was nothing more to see, often the most revealing details would suddenly appear.

This is the way scientific observation works, and it's how emotional connection works too. At first our internal sensations can seem distant and amorphous. But whenever we combine the technique of slowing down with a simultaneous shift into microview, it unearths an entire emotional tableaux.

Gordon described himself as depressed. He walked around feeling distant and cut off from himself and life in general. This condition, he told me during an in-person session, had persisted for decades. It rendered him a chronic underachiever and a refugee from two failed marriages.

I asked Gordon how he knew he was depressed. "I feel like a blob, " he responded. I asked him where in his body that blob was centered. He did a quick scan and pointed to his gut. I directed him to place his attention right there and to notice anything about the blob that he could. Gordon shut his eyes, did his best for a few moments, but then reopened them and shrugged. "It's just a blob, like always," he reported, growing a little frustrated and discouraged.

"Is it warm or cool?" I asked, attempting to prime the pump. He shut his eyes again and checked.

"Neither . . . Well, maybe it's a little warm. Mostly it has kind of a buzzy feeling." Where before there was only vague sensation, now more specific data had begun to emerge. I congratulated Gordon and urged him to keep going. The buzzy feeling, he noticed, spread out to his sides and back. It seemed to move in a clockwise direction. With a little more time Gordon noticed that it grew hot and that his cheeks did as well.

"Now I feel a little scared," he told me. "Out of control." Again I urged him on, suggesting that he get even more microscopic. "Everything just moved to my throat," he said. "But there's a big backup. Like too much energy, and it can't get through. Like I'm about to explode."

I suggested that he keep observing, up close, but with a scientist's even demeanor. He coughed, squinted his eyes. After a few more moments he opened them again. "I'm sad," he said. He looked surprised, almost excited. "Yeah, I feel sad. All over."

For Gordon, connecting to this sadness marked the start of a much longer healing journey. He came to see that his depression had been a defense against a reservoir of long unfelt grief. For our purposes, what's important to highlight is the way that Gordon's perpetual blob, just like an anthill, revealed itself fully under a patient, precise, noninterfering gaze.

2 X 2 PROCESS

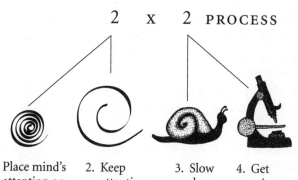

1. Place mind's attention on emotional sensation in body.

2. Keep attention on sensation until it dissipates.

3. Slow down.

4. Get microscopic.

FIGURE 2

Slowing down and getting microscopic is what allows Steps 1 and 2 to create sufficient emotional contact. Steps 1 and 2, in turn, target the exact location necessary for this slow microattention to achieve maximum results. That's why the dual parts of the 2 X 2 process are so interdepedent.* If you completed the exercise on pages 17–18, then you've already laid the foundation for putting this process to use. Back then I asked you to consider whether your physical sensation had an emotional quality, but I didn't provide a specific way to do so. In fact, full application of the 2 X 2 process is the only way. If a physical sensation doesn't feel emotional after a slow microinvestigation, then it almost always isn't.

PRACTICAL TIP

If a physical sensation doesn't seem emotional after a slow microinvestigation, it isn't.

If a sensation is emotional from the outset, or becomes so during such an investigation, then continuing in the same mode is all that's required.

The 2 X 2 process can also help you understand why this distinction between physical sensations with and without emotional aspects is so important. Strictly physical sensations can sometimes be ignored or repressed with no great peril. If you have a sore muscle, for example, there's no need to keep feeling it in order for the muscle to heal. As long as you don't exacerbate the strain, healing will take place whether you're aware it's happening or not.

Emotions, on the other hand, need your direct involvement. They don't need to be felt forever, or obsessively, but just long enough to have their say. When they know that you've really got the message, they disappear. If you don't get the message, however, they stick around and wreak havoc.

---

*Those of you familiar with my earlier work might wonder how the 2 X 2 process compares with the two-question process called *Living the Questions*. They're similar, but the name *2 X 2* emphasizes how our approach to this type of inquiry is as important as the inquiry itself. Also, this new formulation focuses on the primacy of emotions and, therefore, on the physical body where emotions arise.

So let's pause to do the exercise from pages 17–18 a couple more times, now blending in the 2 X 2 process to experience complete emotional connection.

2 X 2 IN ACTION

Place your attention on your body (Step 1). Notice any sensation that stands out. Do you feel something particular in your belly, chest, limbs, or head? Let whatever your attention lands on first be the focus for this exercise. Keep your attention on that sensation for a few moments (Step 2), watching closely to see what happens. Avoid the temptation to influence it in any way.

As you continue to monitor this sensation, remember to Slow Down and Get Microscopic. Does the sensation move or stay fixed? Does it change a little or a lot? Does it lessen or intensify? Or, perhaps, does it seem to remain exactly the same?

See if you can sustain this gentle, inquisitive mode for at least a minute. If your attention wanders or mind chatter begins to take over, just acknowledge what's happening and return to your sensation once again.

At the end of the minute, if you haven't already, notice whether the sensation has an emotional quality. If you don't experience any discernible emotion, just note your overall mood. Perhaps you're calm, energized, curious, pensive, or self-conscious. After noting your mood, bring this first pass of the exercise to a close. Your application of the 2 X 2 process has established that, most likely, no attention-requiring emotions are present.

If you do notice a discernible emotional quality to your experience, extend the exercise for another minute. Rather than trying to understand it, let the emotion reveal itself to you. If a name for the emotion arises, set it aside momentarily so you can keep focusing on the actual experience at hand. If thoughts or realizations about the emotion arise, or about the situation they pertain to, set those aside as well. Continue "surfing" the experience with your attention until the bulk

of its intensity has diminished, or until it has evolved into a different
emotional, or merely physical, sensation.

Whether you did the shorter or extended version of the exercise, pause for a moment and take a few breaths. Reflect on the experience. Was it easy or difficult, strange or familiar? Did it trigger any new or unusual responses? How are you feeling in general about your sojourn into this realm?

Many people find their first few tries at emotional connection somewhat challenging. Fear of the unfamiliar can set off a number of avoidance responses. One of the most common responses is beating a hasty retreat back into thought. This might show up as daydreaming, the sudden need to solve an unrelated problem, or a rapid-fire sequence of random topics that arise for no apparent reason. Another common response is distraction, during which every surrounding sight and sound becomes amplified and insistent, making it seem almost impossible to stay on task.

If any of these responses occurred for you, or if your patience flagged for a different reason, take heart and don't fight it. Instead, let your mind exhaust as many of these avoidance approaches as necessary, calmly returning to the 2 X 2 process as soon as you're able. If you're not able, try again in different moods and at different times of the day. Remember that you're training a "muscle."

PRACTICAL TIP

Learning emotional connection is
like training a muscle.

Just as the same twenty push-ups can seem like a climb up Mount Everest in the morning and then no more than a casual stroll in the afternoon, your degree of ease with emotional connection may vary widely. Even within such variance, however, all muscles do get stronger when worked regularly, and over a surprisingly short period of time. In seeking to strengthen your emotional muscle, don't lose sight of the goal—accessing an incredibly powerful resource that you *already* possess.

Now, before moving on to the second pass of this exercise, we need to revisit something from the first. When I suggested that you set aside any name that arises for your emotion, that's because names often get in the way. They get in the way when we search for them, because the mental activity involved in such labeling can easily pull us out of our direct experience. They also get in the way by taking us out of micromode and into the realm of abstraction.

Strictly speaking, there is no such thing as "happy," "sad," "excited," or "lonely." When we turn to our bodies to find the experiences given those names, what shows up is actually a stream of very specific experiences. "Happy," for instance, may be a warm glow in the chest, or just as easily an all-over tingling. Not only can it be different in different people, but it can also be different for the same person from one occurrence to the next. In addition, the 2 X 2 process reveals that even during a single episode of "happy" the associated experiences can vary widely.

CORE CONCEPT

**Names for emotions are static, while the experience
of them is always varied and dynamic.**

I'm not suggesting that we don't use names for feelings—we'll actually depend upon them greatly in successive chapters—but rather that we recognize these names for the abstractions that they are and then zoom in past them to make tangible emotional contact. Rest assured, when you do make contact, that it works just as well even if you *never* find a name for your feeling.

HEAT OF THE MOMENT

*Taking into account everything from the previous exercise, as well as
the additional instruction about avoidance and labeling, try the 2 X 2*

process of emotional connection again. This time, wait to begin until you're already feeling a strong emotion. This could happen right now, a little later, or sometime in the near future.

The point of the second pass is to gather information about experiencing emotional connection in the heat of the moment. Are you able to maintain your attention, to surf what arises with the same patience and precision as before? If so, stay with the emotion until it's gone or it assumes a significantly different quality. When finished, make note of how the experience was both similar and different from what happened earlier.

If you aren't able to maintain your attention during this more intensive flow, don't worry. What's important is to recognize where and how you lost touch. Did this happen because of avoidance? Did you get sucked under by the power of the emotion and stop witnessing it? Did its intensity cause you to stop short? Or was it something else entirely? This information is invaluable—in a sense it can serve you better than having just cruised through the exercise—since every moment of emotional disconnection shows you exactly where you most need to work the muscle.

By the time you've completed both passes of the above exercise, you'll have put much more than a toe in the water. (Have you noticed that I keep using liquid metaphors? That's because emotional connection really is like surfing most of the time, or swimming, or floating, or diving.) In fact, even if these practice runs went well, you may still feel like you're in a little over your head. The good news is that it doesn't get any more difficult than this, and soon, for the most part, it will get easier.

One reason it gets easier is that your witnessing muscle quickly strengthens, as we already discussed. Another reason is that after you experience a few of the aha insights that only emotional connection can provide, your commitment to the process also strengthens. Still another reason is that fear of the unfamiliar falls away as soon as you visit your feelings more frequently. The "dragon behind the door," to quote one humorous depiction of this transition, "turns out to be a gerbil in drag."

Even with all your growing familiarity and ease, however, there will still be times when emotional connection doesn't flow smoothly. To provide relief during these times, the next chapter introduces several quick, potent methods. After incorporating these methods into your overall approach, we'll move on to a discussion of the habitual ways that most of us disregard our feelings, and how best to stop doing so. At that point you'll be ready to tackle what's holding you back, and to let emotional connection provide your ultimate breakthrough.

~ 4 ~

FROZEN FEELINGS

WHEN YOU HAVEN'T let feelings flow for a while, often there's a backup. Just as with clogged pipes, nothing can get through. Backups also happen when feelings have been flowing, yet suddenly a particular emotion creates a sense of overwhelm. In response to this you may go numb, find it difficult to focus, or experience a kind of hide-and-seek in which the emotion darts away as soon as you draw a bead on it. All these cases yield the same disheartening result—you diligently perform the 2 X 2 process, but nevertheless everything remains frozen.

For these occurrences, the following practices serve both to thaw your emotional system and to let your feelings know that the coast is really clear. Try them one at a time, in any combination, or all at once. Find out which of the group work best for you and under which circumstances. By adding the entire group to your tool kit, you ensure that no emotion will gum up the works for long.*

---

*This comparison of your emotional system to plumbing (more liquid!) isn't just fanciful. New science suggests that many cells in the body have special receptor sites for emotion-related molecules. These receptor sites seem to develop set points that can cling to some emotions and stave off others, creating fixed patterns. The advanced feeling practices in this chapter can function, if you will, as a kind of noncaustic Drano.

Breath

When it comes to stimulating and moving emotion, nothing is more powerful than breath. Breath and emotion impact each one other all the time. Deep breathing, for instance, usually creates a feeling of calm. Fear, when it arises, tends to produce rapid and shallow breath. If emotionally blocked, we can capitalize on this dynamic relationship by breathing *directly into* the area of greatest sensation. This means literally expanding the area with an inhale and then dislodging whatever's stuck by exhaling it out. A series of ten or so breaths taken in this fashion almost always creates renewed flow.

Take a moment to get the hang of it right now. Choose any spot in your body that you'd like to infuse with a little more movement and energy. Place your mental attention on that spot, and breathe into and out of it repeatedly. Slow your breathing to a point that's rhythmic and deliberate yet still natural. Imagine that the current of air inflates and deflates this spot in your body like a balloon. Keep focusing on the spot, performing the 2 X 2 process simultaneously in order to get a detailed view of whatever shifts occur. Continue breathing into the spot until it feels fully fluid.

Breathing into any body part creates inner movement, whether or not emotion is present. It also creates movement even if the spot on which you focus isn't one into which air really enters, such as your fingers or calves. Experiencing this practice when you're not emotionally backed up will help the practice feel more natural when you are.

PRACTICAL TIP

Breathing into an emotion is the opposite of taking a deep breath to escape it.

It's important to note that breathing into an area combines the actual physiological function with a mental visualization of what's happening inside. One without the other is much less effective. It's also important to note that breathing *into* is the complete opposite of taking a deep breath to escape an uncomfortable emotion. Our goal with this practice isn't to avoid or manipulate, but rather to summon the feeling forth so we can welcome it sufficiently.

Posture-Movement-Sound

When an actor prepares for a role, it's customary to work "inside out." This means finding the personal emotions that relate to the character and then letting a repertoire of physical gestures grow from that. Other actors choose to work "outside in," which means starting with all the character's bodily mannerisms and letting them lead the way to analogous emotions. The fact that both approaches can succeed highlights the interplay between feelings and their outward expressions. This recognition is helpful not only for actors attempting to evoke particular emotions, but also for the rest of us when trying to connect with emotions that already exist.

Every emotion that arises in your body has a corresponding posture. If you're angry, it might be natural to make a fist. If you're sad, it might be natural to curl up into a ball. These positions not only express emotion, but they can also liberate it. Therefore, whenever you're emotionally stuck, it's a good idea to assume a posture that's reflective of that very moment. Then, use the 2 X 2 process to see if there's a shift. You don't have to stop there either. It's also possible to stack the deck in your favor by building on what you've already begun.

To do so, let a movement evolve out of your assumed posture. If you're angry, you might shake your fist. If you're sad, you might rock your curled body side to side. These kinds of external movements are especially effective in creating parallel internal movements. Continue them until you notice an emotional unfurling, and change them to match what happens. At a certain point your inner experience will become rich enough to warrant complete focus, and you can let the motion come to a gradual rest.

Sound, though we don't usually think of it as such, is another form of movement. Every sound of significant enough magnitude creates a palpable vibration within your body. Consider what happens when a powerful bass line emits from your stereo speakers—your insides literally tremble. Now, with your lips closed, make the sound "Mmmmmmm." Notice what parts of your body register that specific vibration.

CORE CONCEPT

**Each emotion creates its own unique
internal vibration.**

Continue by making some additional sounds with your mouth both open and closed, and observe the different internal vibrations they create.

Emotions, too, create varying vibrations. These vibrations can be amplified by "sounding" them. Such emotionally related sounds can't be predetermined in a formulaic way, but all you have to do to find the right one in any given moment is just give voice to what you feel. When you do, avoiding words and sticking just to raw sound, you increase the opportunity for any stuck emotion to break loose. If you make the sound along with a matching posture and external movement, the likelihood for release is even greater.

The only thing to keep you from using posture, movement, and sound successfully in freeing up your emotional flow is self-consciousness. For many of us nonthespians it can be downright awkward to "play" our bodies in this way. Yet paradoxically we do it all the time, only unconsciously. Think of how you sit in a chair while attentive (posture). Consider how you fidget while bored (movement). Recall how your tone of voice rises with a case of nerves (sound).

Perhaps this understanding that you're already a pro at what may seem so foreign will allow you to give yourself permission to experiment, to feel momentarily foolish in service of emotional connection and all it brings. One final tip in this regard—if you give it your best shot and still feel too uncomfortable to proceed, try using a mixture of posture, movement, and sound that mirrors the discomfort itself. Demonstrate your own unique expression of utter embarrassment.

Sometimes, this is all it takes to get past even the most daunting initial stiffness. It's good for a laugh regardless, and laughter is a dependable emotional lubricant as well.

Touch

Everyone knows the benefit of touch when it comes to a comforting hug, a pat on the back, a relaxing massage, or an intimate encounter. What all these types of touch have in common is that they come from one person to another. Less well known—and less socially sanctioned—is the power of therapeutic *self*-touch. Such self-touch can be administered in many ways and circumstances, from kneading a pulled muscle to soothing oneself with gentle strokes when stressed. None of these is more potent, however, than using self-touch to assist in emotional connection.

This practice couldn't be more straightforward. When an emotion just won't budge, or won't come fully out of hiding, place your hand upon its current physical location. Leave your hand on this spot to help maintain and deepen your attention and to strengthen the brain-body link. Usually, that's all there is to it. In those moments when this type of touch doesn't coax a reluctant emotion forward, or get a stuck one moving, gently rub the area you're touching as an added encouragement. If the emotion moves, follow it with your touch. Continue in this manner until things are back on track. And if at any time along the way you're not sure where the emotion actually is, place your hand instead upon the part of your body that most forcefully calls your attention.

Direct Inquiry

Whenever a client has difficulty gaining access to a feeling, I ask: "If this emotion could speak, what would it say?" The idea here isn't to figure out the answer but to tune in to the emotion's physical manifestation and, as with a Rorschach test, speak the first thing that comes to mind. If the response comes directly from the emotion, it's always true, at least in a subjective sense. Making the words audible can cause the feeling to stir, and once in motion, it typically stays that way.

I witnessed a dramatic version of this chain of events when spending a little extra time with a workshop participant. Tom was angry, and as we sat together in a classroom after a group session, this anger was locked in his belly like a seething, toxic ball. I guided Tom through all the other advanced practices, but the anger just remained, immovable and uncooperative. On a spontaneous hunch, I asked Tom to go to the chalkboard at the front of the room and write over and over, in big letters, "I'm angry that . . ." completing each sentence with whatever words came to him and reading it out loud as he wrote.

Tom began with a litany of everyday complaints. "I'm angry that my kids don't listen to me. I'm angry that we don't have enough money. I'm angry that my back keeps hurting." Then, with a sudden surge of fury he scrawled, "I'm angry that my mother KILLED HERSELF!"

A few moments of charged silence passed. Visibly shaken, Tom returned to his seat. He told me that he hadn't thought about this incident for a number of years and, after much previous counseling, had considered it behind him. By letting his stuck emotion reveal itself, in its own words, Tom quickly got to the heart of the matter. He not only learned of this old anger's resurgence but also gave it a chance to roar forth and release. The rest of us, by hearing out our emotions in this way, can expect to experience a similar release. That's true whether we're dealing with big issues like Tom's or with the little ones that nag us daily.

Cradling

Most parents instinctively know how to hold a fussy infant. They don't gather it in so close that the child feels pressure to stop crying. Nor do they hold it so far away that the child feels abandoned. There's an in-between spot that's just right, where the baby feels lovingly attended to, but also has as much space as necessary to resolve the distress in its own way.

This is what we mean by cradling. Applied to emotions, it works equally well, especially with the more vulnerable ones. Cradling an emotion, of course, is a mental act. It means temporarily adjusting the quality of your attention from scientific/microscopic to tender/ spacious. While Tom's anger knew just what to say about itself, vulnerable emotions are often nonverbal. Their unwillingness to surface is how they communicate that it's not yet safe enough to do so. Cradling these fragile emotions provides them with that missing safety. Once it's apparent, their longing to be met becomes apparent too. As long as your attention remains cherishing, soothing, even the most timid feelings will soon unveil themselves fully.

Here are two brief vignettes that demonstrate the amazing impact of cradling. The first involved Jordan, a thirty-four-year-old woman about to buy her first house. She found the house, qualified for it, and had both the down payment and the salary to make it a wise purchase. Yet she was too terrified to sign the papers. In using emotional connection to determine what was really going on, Jordan got in touch with a part of herself that felt undeserving of such a nice home. If she'd fought this feeling or tried to reason with it, matters would likely have gotten worse.

Instead, Jordan decided to cradle the undeserving feeling with patience and persistence whenever it surfaced. Her very willingness is what ensured that it only needed to surface a few more times in order to resolve completely. The first time it lasted for about fifteen minutes, and the next two times for about five. This twenty-five-minute investment in advanced feeling was all it took. From that point on, Jordan felt worthy and ready. She signed the papers with relative ease and has lived in the house ever since.

Next there was Barbara, twenty-nine, a perpetual doctoral candidate who'd been stalled on her dissertation for over two years. Like the majority of American women, she had internalized the intense social pressure to be thin. She *was* thin, only to her mind not thin enough. So in yoga class she'd compulsively compare her body to the other participants', and in Manhattan shop windows she'd sneak tortured peaks at her profile. In a phone session, fed up, Barbara broke down and admitted to me that she hated her body. She railed against this hatred as stupid and unfair but also realized it was out of her control.

Guided to cradle the hatred, deciding that she had nothing to lose, Barbara found that in just a few minutes it turned to sadness. This didn't feel much better, but she was relieved to be feeling something different and motivated enough to continue. Cradling the sadness now as a daily practice, she found that it persisted on and off for about a week. Then it began to diminish, and her compulsion diminished as well. Freed of her internal tug-of-war, Barbara felt an upsurge of energy and focus. Finally, as a result, she was able to resume writing her thesis.

In concluding this chapter, it's important to spend a little more time on the often confusing relationship between thoughts and feelings. When you use any of the above methods to connect to your most difficult emotions, you'll also kick up a lot of related thoughts. Together, these thoughts make up the "story" of an emotion. The feeling of rejection, for instance, might be accompanied by the story that "No one will ever love me." This story may include all kinds of evidence from the past to support its assertion. In actuality the story may be right, wrong, or some combination of the two. It may be worthy of further consideration or none at all. But in the heat of the emotional moment no such consideration is advisable. We just don't have the necessary distance. Plus, when feeling our worst, we tend to believe the worst stories and even mistake them for absolute truth. What's more, engaging with stories during emotional connection pulls us right out of the 2 X 2 process and prevents any kind of release.

PRACTICAL TIP

**When stories arise in your mind during emotional
connection, don't get caught up agreeing or
disagreeing with them. Notice them neutrally,
then immediately return to 2 X 2.**

To understand stories better and how to handle them when they arise, let's revisit our last three examples. First came Tom, who used the "Direct Inquiry" technique to get in touch with how angry he still was about his mother's suicide. After this truth was revealed and Tom reconnected with the anger, it wasn't just the emotion itself that took the stage. Tom also noticed a slew of negative thoughts about his mother. A primitive part of him unleashed a story about how selfish and mean-spirited she was, despite the fact that she'd suffered from lifelong mental illness.

I counseled Tom to acknowledge these thoughts every time they surfaced but without responding in any way. The idea was neither to agree nor disagree with the rant, but instead to keep focusing on the raw, physical sensation of the anger. This is precisely what enabled the anger to release. Had Tom let himself be drawn into the story, on the other hand, he would have needlessly kept the anger festering. The story would have continued to fuel the anger—"My mother's behavior justifies it!"—and the anger would have continued to fuel the story—"I wouldn't feel this bad if she weren't so awful!"

Jordan, who cradled her undeserving feelings in order to buy a house, also dealt with a potentially debilitating story. Along with the undeserving feelings came an internal monologue about being spoiled, about not having had to work sufficiently for her money, about how it was immoral to spend so much of that money on shelter when millions in the world went homeless. Monologues like this are sticky, because they may draw upon personal values or make seemingly valid points. But engaging with them during an emotional storm will only lead to cloudy thinking and dubious decision making.

Feel first, think later (introduced in chapter 1) is the best order of focus in such a circumstance. This may seem on the surface like a variation of "count to ten," but it's really the opposite. Our aim isn't to calm down and avoid emotional upset, but instead to feel it all. Usually this provides us with valuable perspective on all those previously irksome thoughts. In Jordan's case, once she cradled the undeserving feeling, the internal monologue quickly quieted. This revealed it to be a mere projection of her passing emotion rather than something she really needed to consider.

With Barbara, the sadness that followed her body hatred spun its own yarn about how she was weak, a loser, unable to resist the media's twisted feminine ideal and therefore nowhere near the independent thinker who could actually complete a Ph.D. By welcoming these thoughts without debate or assent, Barbara literally proved the opposite. Her strength in doing so was what allowed them to pass and was also instrumental in helping her get the degree.

All these examples point to one thing. To perfect the skill of emotional connection, you also have to learn the art of mental detachment. This means being able to notice a train of thought without boarding it, or struggling to derail it. Such a feat is often easier said than done, but with practice the process becomes second nature. Here, to provide a better sense of the actual experience, is a verbal approximation from one of my clients. She journaled the following stream of consciousness while struggling through a painful breakup.

> I feel a pulling sensation in my belly. It seems like loneliness. It makes me want to cry. Now tears are coming. Now I'm having a slew of thoughts, about how I'm never going to find a suitable partner, about how it's my fate, because I don't know how to attract and keep the right kind of person. Wow. That's a heavy verdict. I'm not sure whether I really believe that. I'll take a deeper look later. Right now, though, I'm bringing my attention back to the sensation in my belly. I'm letting the tears continue to come and watching where they take me.

This account of the 2 X 2 process, combined with mental detachment, provides a realistic picture of what happens inside us when we dedicate ourselves to feeling fully. There's a natural and unavoidable back-and-forth movement between feeling and thinking. Sometimes the thoughts go on for a few seconds before you notice them, and other times it takes a minute or longer. Either way, it's crucial to return to the emotions as soon as possible. This is what lets the advanced feeling practices do their job and lets you reap all the benefits.

OBSTACLES TO EMOTIONAL CONNECTION

L ET'S PAUSE FOR A MOMENT to see where we are. At the outset I suggested that the one thing holding you back is resistance to emotion. I posited that this is true regardless of your own specific unfulfilled dreams. I vowed that by mastering the skill of emotional connection and then applying it to your personal situation, you'd experience major breakthroughs.

Next, we began assembling the building blocks necessary for those breakthroughs. The first building block was an overall increase in physical awareness, stemming from a recognition that all emotions arise and pass through your body. The second building block was an increase of receptivity to emotional connection, difficult though the experience often is, which we established by working through the most prevalent arguments against it. The third building block was a short course in precisely how to feel, centered on the 2 X 2 process of initiating connection, staying connected, slowing down, and getting microscopic. The fourth building block was a tool kit for stuck or elusive emotions, containing breath, posture-movement-sound, touch, direct emotional inquiry, and cradling. We rounded out the tool kit by adding mental detachment, a practice necessary for the other tools to function successfully.

With all that in place you might be getting restless. You might be thinking, *I'm now willing and able to feel. You said emotional connection is all I need, so let's get to the dreams-come-true part!* We're almost there, I promise, but a big "boulder" still stands in our way. The boulder is that even when we're willing and able to feel, our instinctive response is not to do it. Only by learning how to overcome this instinctive response can you put everything we've covered to work. This chapter will provide all the instruction necessary. Like the others, it will draw predominantly on your own experience.

We begin with a quick look at the prehistoric mind. While our species has made great strides in the roughly 300,000 years since first evolving, human brains today share the same basic structure and function as that of our ancestors. This means, in essence, that we're not really made for our times. We've created environmental and societal advances faster than evolution can devise the adaptations to match. That's why, for example, many people have an instinctual fear of spiders but not of cars. That's also why we respond in a primitive way to situations requiring a more nuanced approach. Emotional connection is just such a nuanced approach, but it can never stop the primitive one from first occurring.

To use another example from modern life, let's say someone cuts you off on the freeway. Your first response might be to do the same in return, make a rude gesture, or roll down the window and offer a piece of your mind. These behaviors all share the potential of making the situation worse, not better. The fast lane, obviously, is the last place to exact petty revenge. And while a few moments of emotional connection would make this abundantly clear, no amount of it could prevent your primitive response from first occurring the next time you encounter an aggressive driver, at least for a split second.

The primitive response is hardwired. No doubt you've heard it referred to as *fight or flight*. When faced with a saber-toothed tiger, cavemen relied for their survival on choosing between these two options. They also had a third possible response, *freeze*, which could be intentional as in playing dead, or involuntary as in immobilization by terror. All three of these responses were accompanied by bodily changes. These changes affected blood pressure, breathing, perspiration, and overall alertness.

The entire *fight-flight-freeze* apparatus still functions in everyone alive right now. Most of us, of course, are rarely in legitimate life-or-death situations. But the primitive part of the brain doesn't just switch on when it perceives a threat; it also assesses every situation we encounter for its relative blend of safety and danger. It usually errs on the side of caution and can't tell the difference between genuine and imagined peril. If your friend suddenly pretends to punch you, for example, you'll flinch just as in a real fight. Only a few moments later will your reasoning kick in to turn off the alarm.

The primitive part of the brain also doesn't distinguish between internal and external danger. It responds in the same general way to a gunshot as it does to a sharp pain. More important for our purposes, it also perceives any undesired emotion as a threat. When an undesired emotion first arises, the instinctive and protective part of the brain wants it gone, now. It doesn't want us to experience unworthiness, for instance, or resentment. It doesn't understand the purpose of those emotions, only that they feel *bad*.

CORE CONCEPT

The primitive part of your brain can't distinguish between an external threat, such as a gunshot, and an internal threat, such as a painful emotion.

But these emotions originate from the same overall feedback system as the primitive response itself. They're from another part of that system that's also trying to provide us with information. In the first moment of a difficult emotion, therefore, we receive crossed signals. One part of the feedback system wants us to feel, while the other part clearly doesn't.

CROSSED SIGNALS
WHEN EMOTION ARISES

Don't Feel This!   Sadness   Feel This!
Message from   *Message from*
Primitive Brain   *Emotional Center*

FIGURE 3

You might wonder why this is so, since it seems like a glitch in human design. Honestly, I'm not equipped to theorize about such a question, and our mission here is more practical than scientific. What I can say, however, is that these crossed signals draw a comparison to the more lasting predicament of autoimmune disease, in which the body mistakenly turns against itself. The primary result of this confusion, emotionally speaking, is what's best referred to as contraction.

Contraction

When most of us think of contraction, it's in relation to childbirth and the intense effort that's necessary for new life to emerge. Emotional contraction is quite similar, in that we need to get through it in order for our feelings to surface and flow. Rather than reading a lot about contraction, I think it's best that you employ a specialized version of the 2 X 2 process to experience it directly.

Begin by focusing on something that really bothers you. Be courageous and choose a big issue in your life, one that you've struggled with for a long time but still haven't been able to overcome. Perhaps there's a family relationship that just won't heal or a problem related to your work or health. Select a topic that creates intense frustration from the moment you begin focusing on it.

Once you've made your selection, allow all that frustration to flood your body. Next, turn your attention to your body, and notice what happens. Use your developing skill of physical awareness to spot where sensation is primarily arising and to recognize its particular qualities. Is it warm or cool? Heavy or light? Distinct or diffuse? Jagged or smooth? Does it pulse, spin, pull inward, or press outward? Keep going in this way, and then after about a minute relax and shake it out.

Because we're each unique, we each feel contraction in different parts of our bodies and in diverse ways. But the essence of the sensation is remarkably similar for everyone. Contraction is a temporary system lockdown, experienced either as tension (fight/flight) or numbness (freeze). Whether it appears at the temples, the shoulders, the belly, or as an overall discomfort, contraction makes it impossible to connect with whatever emotion is requesting our attention.*

Most of the time, contraction drives that emotion downward into our subconscious. Then the initial physical sensation lessens, and a stalemate ensues. The emotion festers, intensifies, and keeps trying to get us to notice it. The contraction, also now in our subconscious, keeps pushing it down. This ongoing struggle, if prolonged, can create stress, anxiety, depression, illness, and sometimes even death. These are the most damaging effects of emotional *dis*connection.

There's one additional effect, in a category all by itself. As a part of our subconscious, unfelt emotions have an eerie ability to bring into our lives people and situations that force us to feel whatever we originally resisted. This is the source of most negative life patterns. If you refuse to connect with anger, for instance, you'll find yourself persistently encountering the very things that enrage you. If you refuse

---

*As I use the terms, contraction and resistance are similar but not the same. Contraction refers solely to the instinctive, physical, mostly unconscious mechanism by which we attempt to protect ourselves from unwanted emotions. Resistance, which is usually both conscious and unconscious, refers to the state of being that results from contraction. It can persist for just a few minutes, or a whole lifetime.

to embrace insecurity, your most important relationships will keep inducing it. Later we'll discuss this thoroughly, because it's so essential in breaking free of your limitations, but for now let's look at two brief examples.

CORE CONCEPT

**Unfelt emotions bring into your life
people and situations that force you to feel
what you previously resisted.**

Ingrid was a successful fund-raising consultant for some of the nation's largest charities. Her problem was that she just couldn't say no to any client request. Her workload, as a result, was stressful and overwhelming. Despite lots of counseling to reverse this pattern, it escalated over many years to the point of a near breakdown. Together, Ingrid and I determined that the source of this destructive pattern was her fear of disappointing people, and that the emotion such disappointment would produce was unworthiness. The more she tried to stave off unworthiness by saying yes to every request, the more frequent and demanding those requests became. It was as if the outside world was secretly in cahoots with her subconscious. But once Ingrid learned how to allow the feeling of unworthiness and to connect with it directly, she soon grew able to establish healthy workload limits. And her clients, after a brief period of reorientation, simply ceased to be so demanding.

Lynn's negative pattern was in the relationship arena. As if on autopilot, she repeatedly picked demeaning, domineering men. "The names and faces have changed over the years," she recounted ruefully, "but essentially it's the same guy. What he says goes. What I want doesn't count." Each relationship would last until Lynn couldn't stand it anymore, but then she'd quickly, blindly plunge into the next one. The emotion Lynn resisted during all that time, as just one session revealed, was vulnerability. The child of constantly warring parents, she'd learned that it was safest to stay out of the way and keep her own wants and needs to herself. Later in life, as a result, she found it intolerable to have those same wants and needs exposed. But once she reconsidered her aversion to vulnerability and decided to embrace the actual feeling of it, her dating life changed to match. Overbearing men soon lost their allure, and she found herself attracted to more considerate men for the very first time.

Freud, you may recall, theorized about a "repetition compulsion," which causes us to seek out and repeat unpleasant experiences in an attempt to solve, heal, or gain a sense of mastery over them. Emotional connection, it turns out, is the best possible way to accomplish all three. It also, most importantly, eliminates our need to keep repeating.

Whether we call this phenomenon a negative pattern or a repetition compulsion, it only persists as long as we're still contracted against the originally painful emotion. So—how can we cause such contractions to unclench and then proceed with emotional connection as did Ingrid and Lynn? The answer, fortunately, is the same 2 X 2 process that we've been employing all along. With your sustained attention placed directly upon it, every single contraction will soon let go. It may sound outlandish, but that's all it takes. In my hundreds of workshops and client sessions, I've never seen a contraction that wouldn't release. I encourage you to test this for yourself.

You might try it right now, as a matter of fact, if any lingering contraction from the earlier exercise still remains. Even more important, however, is to experiment with this over the next few days whenever you notice that a new contraction has occurred. Most likely, here's what you'll find: not only will the contraction ease, but once that happens, you'll also be able to access the emotion that the primitive part of your brain was trying to protect you from in the first place.

The most significant emotional connection takes place with feelings that you don't like or don't want. Therefore, based on what we've just explored, it will always begin not with the emotion itself but instead with the contraction that it initially elicits. The contraction is both your starting place and your touchstone. As long as you remain connected to it physically, it will lead directly to emotional pay dirt.

Expansion

Now it's time to switch gears and focus on something enjoyable, which you'll soon see provides us with a parallel touchstone.

Begin by thinking of someone or something that lights you up with joy. This could be a young child, a place in nature, a pet, or perhaps a favorite activity or memory. Whatever it is, make sure that just to reflect upon it creates an automatic inner smile. Once you've made your selection, allow all that positive energy to permeate you completely. Next, turn your attention to your body, and notice what you feel. Where, mostly, do you feel the sensation? Is it warm or cool? Heavy or light? Distinct or diffuse? Jagged or smooth? Does it pulse, spin, pull inward, or press outward? After a minute or so conclude the exercise and return to ordinary awareness.

What you've just experienced is expansion. As both the name and exercise make clear, it's the opposite of contraction. No matter where or how expansion shows up within each of us, its essence is always a quality of openness and flow. It coexists naturally with positive emotions, like the joy we used to evoke it in this exercise, but it can also coexist with any emotion. In fact, what I meant by calling it a touchstone is that emotional connection of any kind *produces* expansion. If you become expanded, you can trust that you're successfully connected.

PRACTICAL TIP

The presence of expansion indicates successful emotional connection.

And usually, at that point, any key insights carried by your emotion have already been delivered. Do you recall I said earlier that the goal of feeling is to stay connected with an emotion until it either dissipates or changes? Another way to look at it is that expansion is the natural endpoint. You're free to remain in close connection after expansion occurs, but it's usually not necessary.

Rarely do we experience complete expansion, or complete contraction. Complete expansion is akin to what's referred to colloquially as "the zone." Complete contraction might best be described as a whole-body migraine. They're each at either end of a continuum. Toward the center of the continuum are similar but less marked states. A more ordinary degree of expansion feels like a quiet harmony with yourself and the world. A more ordinary degree of contraction feels like being off, or out of sorts. The more aware you become of this whole continuum, the easier it is to spot and unravel all types of contraction quickly. This, in turn, frees you to live more consistently in an expanded state.

Compulsion

None of us, however, is in touch bodily 100 percent of the time. Therefore, it's helpful to have another sign that contraction is afoot. That sign is compulsive behavior. Anything you do compulsively—such as eating, shopping, having sex, watching TV, Web surfing—is a sign of contraction. To be more accurate, it's *caused* by contraction. These behaviors are outer manifestations of your inner-system overload. They're attempts to alleviate the discomfort, which often work in the short term but never over the long haul. On the other hand, as soon as you connect emotionally in any given moment, you alleviate the discomfort at the source, and therefore the compulsion soon diminishes.

As usual, I don't expect you to take my word for it. The next time you feel that itch for your compulsive activity of choice, instead of scratching it right away, pause briefly instead. During that pause locate the corresponding contraction in your body (it will always be there) and proceed to emotional connection. Continue until you're expanded, then reassess the compulsion's strength. Almost always you'll find it gone. In its absence you'll be able to make a much more conscious decision about whether or not to engage in the original activity. Plus, if you do decide to go ahead with it, the result will be much more enjoyable.

Before continuing, I want to explain why, in the last two paragraphs, I didn't use the word "addiction" to describe the habitual behaviors caused by contraction. That's because most people don't suffer from such a full-blown medical condition and certainly don't identify themselves as sick. Yet virtually every one of us acts compulsively from time to time. Rather than signs of illness, these compulsions can be considered *opportunities* for emotional connection. Later, in chapter 11, we'll look at specific cases where the presence of a powerful addiction or compulsion was precisely what provided the road map to personal breakthrough.

To this point, we've broadened our overall picture of emotional connection to include the contraction that accompanies an unwanted feeling. We've also added the expansion that ensues once we penetrate such a contraction and proceed long enough with our 2 X 2 process. We've seen how, along with contraction, a compulsive urge of any kind is another important emotional heads up. Now, in concluding our look at the obstacles to emotional connection, we need to focus on what happens *after* connection has commenced.

As discussed in the previous chapter, our thoughts, beliefs, and stories prevent emotional connection from proceeding without interruption. Most of us are able to apply our attention to feelings only in fits and starts. No problem with that, as long as we keep going. But there can also arise a related type of hindrance in the mental approaches we bring *to* emotional connection. Specifically, the following four impediments are what we need to identify, understand, and defuse.

Analyzing

What analyzing means, in this context, is that instead of connecting straightforwardly to an emotion that's arising, we also try to figure out *why* it's arising. Underlying our urge to analyze is a belief that figuring out an emotion will make it go away. This adds a layer of resistance to our efforts that usually makes them backfire. Because the emotion isn't fully embraced, it just sticks around and waits.

To be sure, the capacity for analysis is one of the great features of the human brain. But when analyzing happens before emotional connection has been sufficiently established, it can't be trusted. It becomes another kind of compulsion and only serves to reinforce our contraction. Plus, analyzing stymies the deeper understanding that emotional connection often provides.

Analyzing can occur at the contraction stage, as in *Why do I suddenly feel so tense?* It can occur at the beginning of the emotional connection stage, as in *There's a flutter in my chest. I get it—I'm nervous. What do I have to be so nervous about?* It can also occur at later stages, as in *Man, I've been connecting to this nervousness for a whole five minutes. Why isn't it going away?*

In all these cases, the way to defuse analyzing begins with becoming aware of it. This draws upon the mental detachment discussed earlier, and specifically the ability to detach from your thoughts long enough to recognize them for what they are. With analyzing, the tip-off is usually a dissatisfied, probing quality—it's as if the thoughts themselves have a furrowed brow, whether you actually do or not. As soon as you notice that you're analyzing, the next step is simply to accept that it's been happening. This is equally true whether it's been happening for a few seconds or a few days.

PRACTICAL TIP

All four impediments are types of resistance. Resisting their presence only creates more resistance. Accepting an emotion, on the other hand, defuses the hindrances instantly.

What's crucial is that your acceptance comes without self-criticism, blame, or any other kind of resistance that will just serve to make you tenser. Translated into words, the effective version of acceptance might come out something like this: *Oh, look. I've been analyzing.* There's a calm, uncomplicated quality to this recognition. The ineffective version, by contrast, might go something like this: *Damn! I'm analyzing again! Why do I keep doing that?!* Did you catch, in this example, how easy it is to heap analyzing upon analyzing? Whenever that happens, or anything else happens to keep you stuck in analyzing mode, simply note it in the effective manner demonstrated above, and you'll be back on track. Once you are, all that's left is to return your attention to the original sensation. Whether it's still the same or has shifted, your emotional connection can now continue.

Judging

When judging, instead of aiming simply to connect with our emotional experience, we decide that there's something wrong with it. We view the emotion as a problem, as something that's not supposed to be happening. Most of the time, judging is accompanied by the words "should" and "shouldn't." We catch ourselves having thoughts like *I shouldn't be feeling this way*, or *I shouldn't let him get to me*, or *I should be over this already.* Along with judging comes a desire to get out of the feeling rather than into it, to change our experience before really engaging with it. As you can see, this renders judging another flavor of resistance and therefore prevents us from reaping the rewards of our emotional exploration.

Fortunately, we can defuse judging in exactly the same way as analyzing. First we become aware of it, next we calmly accept that it's been occurring, and then we return our inward gaze to the raw, unmediated physical sensation that gave rise to it. But judging emotions is especially hard to shake because often we also judge ourselves for having the feeling and thus add guilt or unworthiness upon the situation. Just as it's possible to heap analyzing on analyzing, we can all too easily heap feelings *about* feelings on top of one other. This doesn't release the original feelings—it only obscures them. It can then take a little extra time to deconstruct the pyramid of resistance that we've built. That's why, alongside the other tools in our toolbox, it helps to add a hearty dose of patience. The ability not to take ourselves too seriously also goes a long way.

Assessing

All of us, it seems, have an assessing function that keeps tabs on how well we're doing with whatever task is at hand. That's natural, helpful even, except during the types of activities that we must *relax into* and therefore temporarily suspend our vigilance. Emotional connection, obviously, is one of those activities.

During emotional connection, assessing usually occurs whenever we start wondering if we're "doing it right." Often that wondering progresses to a paralyzing self-doubt, and all is temporarily lost. When assessing, you might notice additional thoughts like *I only keep connecting to my back pain—where's the emotion?* or *Am I supposed to be this distracted?* or *All I can sense is some vague agitation—maybe emotions just aren't my thing.* In cases like these, just as with analyzing and judging, awareness and acceptance are key. As soon as we become aware of and accept our assessing, we're able to resume the 2 X 2 process with no harm done.

Bargaining

Bargaining is the subtlest of the four impediments. It occurs when we recognize that emotional connection is the fastest way through a difficult passage of feeling. We therefore pursue it with that goal in mind. Yet in order to work, emotional connection must be goalless. As soon as our minds fix on a desired result, we're a little less attentive to what's happening right now. On the contrary, whenever we dive into emotional connection for its own sake, without needing to get something out of it, our attention deepens. As a result, that's when we *do* get the most out of it.

If we start putting time limits on how long we're willing to connect to an emotion, that usually signals bargaining. Likewise, when we pretend to give the 2 X 2 process our all but aren't really invested fully, that signals bargaining too. Because it's a subtle state, no one else can tell for sure whether or not you're bargaining. It even takes a little time to develop your own bargaining detector. However, an ability to be honest with yourself is all that's required. In those moments when you're stuck and the tool kit isn't helping you get things moving, simply ask: *Am I bargaining?* Then just be patient and let the answer arise. If the answer is no and doesn't come with a defensive edge, trust it and resume connecting. If it's yes, simply accept that you've been bargaining, and then rededicate yourself to complete connection.

With the added information about *fight-flight-freeze,* contraction, and compulsion, you're equipped to recognize and understand the instinctive choice not to feel. Having explored expansion, you also know how to tell when this instinct is successfully overcome. Finally, in learning about the four impediments of attitude—analyzing, judging, assessing, and bargaining—you've acquired the ability to overcome them too.

The only additional requirement for you to master emotional connection as a lifetime practice is just that- practice. Gradually, as you grow more skillful in solo emotional connection, you'll also be able to employ it while interacting with others. In later chapters we'll revisit this topic, and you'll learn how to bring the 2 X 2 process to bear during conflicts and crises, right in the heat of the moment when most people get lost in unconscious reactivity.

As an added benefit, your communication will improve. You'll have the capacity, during challenging times, to get to the heart of the matter rather than circle it superficially. What's more, the ability to connect with yourself emotionally will also help you tune in to the emotions of others, often before, and even better than they can. This will increase your effectiveness as a friend, family member, partner, coworker, and leader. There's virtually no aspect of your life that won't improve when you approach it with a greater degree of emotional connection.

But the focus of this book, as you know, is more specific. It's about using emotional connection to break through in the area of life where you're most motivated to heal, change, grow, or succeed. All the necessary pieces are now in place for you to do just that. So next, in part 3, I'll explain exactly how.

PART THREE

BREAKING
THROUGH

~ 6 ~

FIND THE FLINCH

Annette was an office manager in Rhode Island. Her secret wish had always been to start a flower-arranging business for weddings. For almost two years she'd had all the information necessary to begin but hadn't done a single thing with it. In fact, she now avoided her home office entirely.

I asked Annette to imagine herself in the office doorway, about to enter and get to work. Immediately, she reported feeling "scared to death," with a huge lump in her throat.

"Scared of?" I asked.

"Hmm. You know, I thought it would be fear of failure, but what's coming up is something different." Annette went on to describe a legacy from her childhood in which she learned to be seen and not heard. Putting herself forward without being asked was always met with such fury that she quickly learned never to do it. Starting a new business, therefore, felt like trying to get away with something.

When her fear subsided a bit, I asked Annette to tell me the worst thing that could happen if she went ahead and started the business anyway. "Well, I'm not sure," she replied. "I've never thought that far ahead."

Hearing this, I painted a purposely dire scenario. I suggested Annette imagine that her business was up and running and that she delivered a floral arrangement to a client who was angry and disappointed, shouting, "Who do you think you are to bring me this?! You don't even *deserve* to be a florist!"

Annette seemed to shrink. She said that her chest and shoulders felt wrapped up like a mummy. I asked her to keep her attention on all that tightness, to regard it with as much space and tenderness as possible.

"It's starting to release," she told me after a few moments. "Now I feel humiliated, like I'm being punished for the whole world to see."

"Keep feeling that too," I encouraged, knowing she'd struck gold. Annette's unwillingness to feel this humiliation had been the one thing holding her back. Next, to break through, all she needed was to stay fully connected to the humiliation. She did so, bravely, and after about three minutes it began to subside. Relieved, Annette was also a little stunned.

"Wow. That wasn't as bad as I thought." I remained silent for a while to let all this register. Then I asked her how, from this place of relaxation and acceptance, she would respond to the disappointed client.

"I guess . . ." She paused for the truest answer to emerge. "I guess I could just apologize and see if there's a way to fix the problem."

This simple recognition was the beginning of Annette's personal transformation. It was also the beginning of her business. Shortly afterward she began going to trade shows and making cold calls. Soon, she was handling between two and three weddings a month.

Within this brief account exists a formula to break through the one thing holding *you* back. The best way to draw out that formula is by walking through Annette's experience a second time, inserting additional details and viewing it through the framework constructed earlier. We'll begin the walk-through here and continue it for the next three chapters. Once you've read through them, consult the formula diagram on page 91 for easy reference.

Annette had a specific and tangible goal. She'd begun to pursue it and then became powerfully blocked. When she told me that she avoided her home office, I knew there was an actual location connected to this block. I asked Annette to focus on that location, in her mind's eye, because doing so was a quick and surefire way for her to experience the block in the present and to recognize its physical nature. The physical nature of any block is the contraction that we covered in the previous chapter. It's what occurs when our primitive brains are threatened by an unwanted emotion. This reflex to fight, flee, or freeze in response to the emotion shows up primarily as bodily tension or numbness. The first step necessary to enable emotional connection—what I call "find the flinch"—is bringing this contraction to light

In addition to evoking a location, as Annette did, there are other equally potent ways to find the flinch in relation to your goals. You can focus on a dreaded conversation, a particularly difficult person, or any significant action with which you've been struggling. This struggle may take the form of avoidance, like Annette's, but it may also appear as lack of follow-through or consistency. Or you may have managed complete follow-through and consistency yet still met with demoralizing setbacks.

No matter which is true for you, find the flinch means recognizing the moment that you ordinarily seize up or check out in relation to your goal.

CORE CONCEPT

Find the flinch means recognizing how you seize up or check out in pursuit of your goal.

You'll know you're on the right track because of the contraction that results. If you don't contract, experiment with other potential "flinchers" until the effect is as uncomfortable as it is unmistakable.

Before we move on, let's see how the flinch occurs in situations when the goal is more modest. At work, you may want a raise but contract every time you imagine bringing it up with your boss. Or you may have an idea for how to solve a problem but shy away from sharing it because of all the naysayers in your department. At home, you may cringe at the thought of disciplining your child because of the tantrum that usually results. Or you may shut down sexually with your partner because of a simmering hurt that's too difficult to express. What unites all these examples is that you're prevented from reaching the goal because a contraction repeatedly stops the show.

In the previous account of contraction, I described it as what happens when our brains, simultaneously, signal us both to feel and avoid feeling. The same effect is also created when we *imagine* feeling an emotion in the future. In the process a bit of that emotion gets elicited by our imagining. This emotional tremor, no matter how small, is still enough to shut us down.

PRACTICAL TIP

**Imagining how you'll feel about something
that hasn't yet occurred can create a contraction
similar to the actual experience.**

So whether our flinch arises frequently in regard to work, home, or anything else, over time it becomes a kind of mind/body habit, a system set point that can rarely be reasoned with or overcome by will. That's precisely why we feel so stuck.

With an understanding of what's involved in a flinch and how to find yours, let's return to Annette. Her flinch showed up as a lump in the throat and also the feeling of being "scared to death." Often, along with the other aspects of contraction that we've covered, there's also a corresponding fear. Sometimes the two come simultaneously, and sometimes one follows the other. Either way, fear is a phenomenon that now requires a closer look.

Just as anxiety is usually a feeling about a feeling, so, too, is fear. Most of the time it's an additional part of our survival response, designed to help keep us from experiencing other emotions. We find ourselves, for example, reacting with a surge of adrenaline to hurt, grief, anger, or loneliness, as if they were footsteps in a darkened alley. We instinctively fear that these emotions will be too painful or overwhelming. On a primal level it seems like they'll kill us, or turn out to be a fate *worse* than death. Even once we're adept enough at emotional connection to know this isn't true, we're still likely to go through that same initial reaction. Along with that reaction, inevitably, comes the mistaken assumption that agreeing to feel a scary emotion right now will doom us to feel it forever or at least for way longer than we're willing (see appendix A, pages 194–198).

What all this means is that in order to connect with many emotions directly, we must first use the 2 X 2 process to move through the fear of them.

PRACTICAL TIP

To establish connection with many emotions requires first moving through the fear of them.

Fear has a unique tendency, once given the chance, to create a kind of flash flood. For a few drenching moments it can seem like we're truly no match for its intensity. Yet with practice we come to see that the flood almost always subsides quickly. Then, in its wake, we're free and clear to connect with whatever emotion had attempted to get our attention in the first place.

In rare cases this doesn't happen, and the fear persists for more than a couple of minutes. Sometimes that's because we're temporarily too fragile or stressed for the kind of attention and resilience that emotional connection requires. Here it's important to heed the fear as a genuine warning and wait for a better opportunity. Other times the fear persists because our current distress has stirred up a residue of serious past trauma. Here, too, it's best to hold off and also to seek the support of a qualified counselor.

There's one more circumstance when fear persists, and that's if the emotion we need to connect with *is* the fear. Some people have more trouble tolerating fear than any other feeling. I once worked with such a man, Michael, under the glare of bright lights in a television studio.

Michael suffered from a severe fear of commitment. It kept him from most second dates, let alone relationships. During our videotaped session I assisted Michael in embracing this fear slowly and steadily, one moment at a time via the 2 X 2 process. The fear caused him to pale, tremble, and dart his eyes around the room like a trapped animal. To his great credit Michael stayed with the process for a full five minutes. Then, suddenly, he relaxed. His color returned, the trembling stopped, and he looked straight at me with bemused calm.

It was a revelation to Michael that there was any existence at all on the other side of his paralyzing terror. This discovery left him grateful and cautiously willing to experiment with further intimacy. But when the cameras were off, and no one else was within earshot, he confessed that the only thing that kept him seated during the strongest waves of fear was the microphone cord taped to the floor and then fed up through his sweater. Had he not been so restricted, Michael sheepishly told me, he'd have been out the door and blocks away before anyone even knew what happened.

$$\sim \quad 7 \quad \sim$$

CUT TO THE CHASE

O NCE YOU FEEL WELL ENOUGH in touch with whatever contraction and/or fear is present, it's time for the next step. I call
this step "cut to the chase," because it's designed to quickly dispense
with any and all distracting stories about the issue. Here's how it works:
ask yourself, *What's the worst thing that could happen if I went forward
beyond my flinch?* Rather than jumping to conclusions, let the answer
come on its own. When it has, follow up with the companion question,
If this worst-case scenario did happen, how would it make me feel? Let
this answer come on its own as well, without any struggle. Look for it—
where else?—in your body.

Usually the answers to these questions come quickly and clearly. With
Annette, they didn't. But because we knew her fearful response brought
up echoes of trying to get away with something as a child, the direction to
explore was clear. If you ever get stuck cutting to the chase and are looking
for direction, it's a good idea to explore your own past for highly charged
situations similar to the flinch that you're working with currently. (For
more on such "emotional association," see pages 142–143).

Sometimes, when asking these Cut-to-the-Chase questions, the
answer is strong but not specific. If stalled in asking for a raise, to return

to a previous example, you might know precisely the worst thing that could happen. "My boss would laugh in my face," you might reply. But contemplating how you'd feel, you might come up with something like, "I'd freak out," or "I'd just die." It's obvious that these statements aren't literal and also that they belie some seemingly intolerable emotional fallout. A little more information here is important. The information you're looking for is visceral though not conceptual. So when encountering these exaggerated replies, it's useful to add such physically oriented follow-ups as, *What would freaking out actually feel like?* and *Where would I experience that in my body?* As always, let your answers to these questions rise to the surface in their own way and time.

The answers that inevitably do arise are finite in number. While their combinations and shadings may be many, the most commonly avoided emotions are relatively few. Here's a list:

anger	sadness	weakness
disappointment	loneliness	despair
hurt	distrust	boredom
rejection	jealousy	insecurity
resentment	longing	pressure
hatred	stress	hopelessness
confusion	shyness	disgust
shame	self-consciousness	unworthiness
humiliation	overwhelm	abandonment
fear	grief	love
vulnerability	guilt	happiness

Take some time to consider this list. How many of the emotions do you definitely avoid? How many do you possibly avoid? Which one or two do you avoid the most? Is one that pertains to you missing? Whenever you encounter an unpleasant emotion that's not on this list, it's almost certainly related to one that is.

In case you're not sure of the answers to these questions, here's a brief inquiry to help you find out.

1. Name three people from your work world, present or past, to whom you've had a harsh negative reaction.

_____

_____

_____

2. Name the most objectionable quality of each person.

_____

_____

_____

3. One at a time, conjure each individual in your mind's eye, exhibiting his or her objectionable quality. Then use the 2 X 2 process to identify how this quality makes you feel. Record your findings below.

_____

_____

_____

If you get more than one response to a single quality, include them all. Spend enough time in seeking your responses to get past the initial contraction and/or fear that's likely to arise with each quality. You know you haven't broken through to the actual emotion yet if all you come up with are synonyms for "irritated." If you do spend considerable time and still don't get a distinct emotional response, repeat the exercise, and heighten the objectionable quality in your mind's eye to an almost absurd extreme.

Next, perform the same inquiry with the three most problematic people in your family, relatives included. Do it, in addition, for the three people who annoy you the most among your friends and social network. Try it with public figures, too, like celebrities and politicians. Finally, substitute three difficult people with three situations you can't bear, such as being falsely accused or making a huge gaffe in front of your peers.

The emotions you've encountered during the above inquiry are undoubtedly some of the same ones you resist the most. We can draw that conclusion because strong negative reactions to people and situations are almost always emotionally based. If you didn't resist the feeling of unworthiness, for example, then you wouldn't be so vexed by that manager who's quick to call you on your mistakes. If you didn't resist the feeling of jealousy, then you wouldn't have such a knee-jerk aversion to your best friend's new confidant.

A key principle, worth restating, is that resistance to emotion is what causes the majority of trouble for all of us. It's what impedes us from our greatest triumphs. The above list and inquiry make this principle more tangible. *An ability to feel those thirty-three physical states consciously, without shutting down, whether able to name them or not, until reaching a state of expansion, would make a colossal difference in your life.* It would also provide a powerful advantage in reaching any of your important goals.

Furthermore, recognizing the emotions that other people in your life have difficulty feeling is also an invaluable skill. Think of the people you deal with most often. Take another look at the list, and see if you're clear or even have a strong hunch about which emotions provide the greatest difficulty for these individuals. If you're not clear on this, you're likely to stumble when collaborating with or confronting them. If you are clear, you'll usually be able to get your point across or advance your objectives without triggering them unnecessarily to fight, flee, or freeze.

Let's also pause to consider the last two emotions on the list: love and happiness. You may question that such "positive" emotions would be avoided. Yet at all my workshops they come up. Almost always, the reason people give for this avoidance is, "I don't deserve to feel that way." In these cases, self-judgment is so powerful that it even causes contraction against the feeling states that are most pleasurable.

8

WEATHER THE STORM

ONCE YOU'RE AWARE of the worst-case scenario and how it would make you feel, the next step is to imagine that all this has actually come to pass. Visualize the situation in all its awfulness, and then give yourself completely to the resulting internal experience. Your imaginary version is never the same as the real thing, of course, but it's almost always enough to create emotional connection, which is really all we're after.

For some people it's easier to sink into the scenario than others. If it's a little difficult for you, take extra care to tease out the scenario's details. What time of day is it occurring? Is it cloudy outside or clear? Pay special attention to the realm of the senses—the tone of people's voices, the style of their clothes, any scent in the air, the taste in your mouth, and those hairs that may be standing up on the back of your neck.

You know you've done your imaginary work when it registers physically. You don't have to dream it up anymore because now you feel it. And if you lose the thread of feeling at any point along the way, just take a moment to flesh out the situation again, or revisit the first blast of emotional impact in the story you're evoking. With all that, if you still have difficulty stirring up a storm in order to weather it, practice on a powerful memory.

When I was in seventh grade, for instance, I did one of the stupidest things in my life. The door had just been painted in my wood-shop class, and while it was still wet, a pal suggested we carve our initials into it. That seemed harmless and anonymous enough, so I joined him gleefully, never stopping to think that to find the culprits, our teacher simply needed to scan through all his roll books. Needless to say, I was soon busted and did some serious time in detention. I didn't mind the punishment, but the dim-witted nature of my crime made me cringe with utter shame. All I have to do still, three decades later, is picture those hastily scrawled initials, and a wave of the same shame roars through me.

Which of your own significant memories, to this day, still have the power to induce waves of emotion? It doesn't matter whether those emotions are enjoyable or painful, only that you let them wash over you now. Calling upon the past in this way will almost always strengthen your ability to do the same with your worst-case scenario.

When Annette envisioned the worst-case scenario of furious and demeaning clients, instead of attaining emotional flow as a result, she first contracted like a "mummy." It took a few moments of 2 X 2 before she landed dead center in a storm of humiliation. This recontraction, following her initial flinch, is in keeping with everything we've discussed about our instinctive response to unwanted emotion. While weathering the storm, we temporarily push ourselves to experience a feeling that our primitive brains consider a mortal foe. We can never bypass the fight, flight, or freeze that follows but only work our way through it. And even when we do, some contractions are still bound to grip us again, often when we think we're well beyond them. That's why a back-and-forth movement between feeling and contracting is normal and nothing to worry about, as long as our overall trajectory is a deepening of connection.

Once Annette was in full feeling, what was it she actually felt? At the time, she and I both called it humiliation, but we also let the 2 X 2 process work its magic. Turning her attention to her body, she felt a sick feeling deep in the belly. Leaving her attention there, she felt that sick feeling vault to her cheeks and turn them red hot. Slowing her attention down brought on a minute of tears. Getting microscopic sent her back to the original sick feeling in her belly, which now took the form of a marble, but then quickly dissolved ("Like Alka-Seltzer," she told me) and led directly to her expansive relief.

PRACTICAL TIP

When weathering the storm, it's natural to experience a back-and-forth between feeling and contracting.

Total elapsed time—about three minutes. Yet the resulting change was life altering, and here's why: Humiliation had been Annette's nemesis. The more she resisted it, the more it pushed back. The more it pushed back, the more energy it took to suppress. This vicious cycle was not only painful and debilitating, but it also backfired. The screeching halt it brought to her dream actually served to *create more humiliation!*

That's how it always happens. An unfelt emotion inevitably wins, sabotaging all our best efforts until we finally invite it onto the team. Once we connect with it, however, the emotion holds no grudge and exacts no revenge. It makes the process no more difficult than it has to be. Instead, it leads us directly into a state of expansion, which is right where we need to go.

What makes this practice so powerful is that *you're retraining your brain not to label the emotion as a threat.* You now know that the worst-case scenario and its resulting emotion are bearable after all. You know this from direct experience. Therefore, your brain doesn't need to stay in permanent contraction to avoid it. Even if you still do contract from time to time, you're able to notice it and bring about a quick release. The emotion may be unpleasant, but you simply accept it as part of your natural feedback system, connect to it, and ride it through to expansion. This approach to your emotional life creates the greatest possible well-being. It also, as we're about to see, does far more than that.

Earlier, we looked briefly at how our thoughts are not trustworthy while we're contracted. We noted that if we're contracted, thoughts that *seem* rational and appropriate to a given situation are actually designed to avoid a feeling. This means our creative powers are limited and distorted whenever we're not willing to feel. Now, let's take that topic further.

Like most writers, I procrastinate. As soon as it's time to sit down at my computer, suddenly I realize all the things that have to be done around the house. There are dishes that need washing, refrigerator shelves that need reorganizing, plants that are crying out for water, and windowsills that simply must be dusted this very minute!

What's tricky about this situation is that all those tasks are real and necessary. My mind is able to make a compelling case in such moments that the writing can wait, or that these other projects are good writing warm-ups, or that it's time to give myself a break and stop being such a slave driver. If I trusted these trains of thought and followed them into action, I'd succeed at being a good housekeeper while letting my writing goals fall by the wayside. While they're certainly rational, these thoughts are not at all in my best interest. They're actually part of the ingrained mechanism we've been discussing that's designed to keep me from feeling.

How do I know that? Because I've learned, every time they appear, to turn my attention to my body. And what I always find is a contraction. So I ask myself, *What's the worst thing that could happen if I sat down at my computer right now, and how would it make me feel?* The answer is usually something like, *No words would come, and I'd feel restless, surly, and frustrated.* So then I weather the storm until I reach an expanded state.

At that point I realize that it's okay to feel restless, surly, and frustrated and that I'll get through it. I realize that writing is a higher priority for me than windowsill dusting and that such dusting can happen at other times when I have less quality energy available to put toward my writing. I also realize that if I dust a few windowsills on the way to my computer, it won't be the end of the world. But no, I don't need to do that right now.

So I sit down to write. And no words come. I feel restless, surly, and frustrated. I ache for a distraction, an escape, and of course my superfast Internet connection is full of them. If I'm on my game, though, I recognize that ache as a temporary recurrence of contraction and use the 2 X 2 process to open back up and weather this *actual* storm just as I've weathered the previous imaginary one. Next, I just sit there for a while, peaceful and expanded, staring at the blank screen. Then, sometimes slowly, sometimes in a flurry, the words begin to come.

There's one part of the above description that may seem a bit ridiculous. You may think that those procrastinating thoughts about housework are obviously bogus and easy to overcome without all the additional emotional work. Similarly, you may have thought that it was obvious how Annette could successfully handle a potentially irate client without having to go through such a torrent of humiliation. But the hallmark of contracted thinking is a massive, impenetrable blind spot. Even though the rest of the world might be able to see a situation clearly, while contracted, we simply can't. This is not just true for individuals, but also for groups of any size.

Once weathering the storm removes such blind spots, of course there's still lots of work to be done in bringing about our goals. If we don't do that work, for whatever reason, we'll fail anyway. Plus, even if we do the work, there are plenty of other factors entirely out of our control that may trip us up regardless.

To reiterate, emotional connection is not a quick fix or shortcut. It will, however, dramatically improve our efforts both in the short term and over the long haul.

For those of you who would appreciate a conceptual foundation for this claim, let's conclude this chapter by turning our attention back to the brain. Neuroscience has shown us that the brain has three basic levels. At the core is our primitive survival system, home of the fight-flight-freeze response we've already discussed in detail. Surrounding the primitive brain is the limbic system, which primarily governs memory and all emotional responses besides survival-based fear. Surrounding the limbic system is the neocortex, which gives rise to our abstract reasoning. The scientist who first created and applied this model was Paul MacLean. He called it the "triune brain" (see figure 4).*

Evolution developed this triune brain, in order, from the most simple to the most complex. Complex does not always trump simple, however, and for their most fruitful functioning these three parts of our brains must constantly work together. In fact they rely upon one another.

When that interdependence breaks down, contraction is almost always the culprit. Therefore, in order to regain full function, we need to attend to ourselves in evolutionary order. What I mean is this: Only when a contraction releases can we feel our emotions. And only when we've felt our emotions can we think clearly. If we try to feel without first releasing a contraction, it won't work. If we try to think clearly without first connecting emotionally, that won't work either (see figure 5).

Among our attempts to outwit evolution, one stands apart. That's when we employ our thoughts out of order specifically to "handle" feelings. Does this sound familiar? It mostly takes the form of analyzing, judging, and bargaining. But it also pertains to thinking about feelings *without*

THE TRIUNE BRAIN

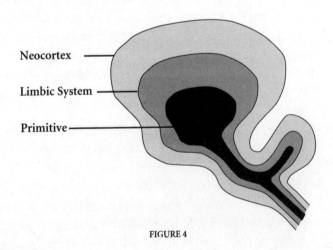

Neocortex

Limbic System

Primitive

FIGURE 4

---

*MacLean originally called the oldest part of the brain "R Complex," referring to its reptilian origins. I've taken the liberty of retitling it to make his point more descriptive.

trying to get rid of them, which we haven't yet discussed. We may do this alone, in one-on-one conversation, or in groups. It may take the form of journal writing, therapy, or even a staff meeting. No matter how or where it occurs, such out-of-order thinking is often hard to spot because it seems so emotion friendly. After all, emotions are indeed the topic.

Yet thinking about emotions and feeling them are very different experiences. They also lead to very different results. Thinking about emotions before feeling them creates the illusion that we've already accessed the emotions in question and therefore lessens our likelihood to double back and connect directly. To connect with an emotion effectively, therefore, requires that we postpone the majority of our thinking about it until after the prior two evolutionary steps are accomplished (see figure 6).

There are, of course, exceptions to this rule. One exception is when thinking helps identify an emotion that needs to be felt. As long as we then go on to 2 X 2 with the emotion itself, no worries there. Another

INEFFECTIVE ATTEMPTS TO ADDRESS EMOTIONS

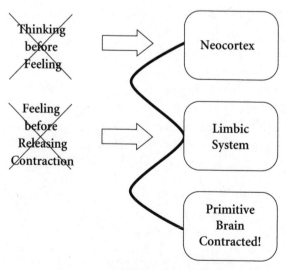

FIGURE 5

EVOLUTIONARY ORDER FOR ADDRESSING EMOTION

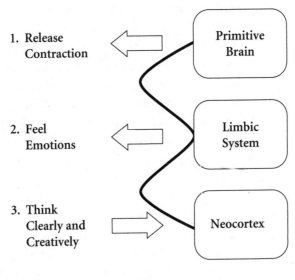

FIGURE 6

exception is when thinking about a feeling actually elicits it. This allows us the chance, right in the moment, to switch gears and connect. The third exception regards those brief excursions of thought that almost always accompany emotional connection.

But these exceptions prove the rule. They help us remain ever flexible while recognizing the majority of times that we mistakenly prolong or intensify emotions with our well-meaning tendency to muse and chat about them. It turns out that "Feel first, think later" isn't just a commonsense maxim—it also derives from the origin of our species.

~ 9 ~

REPEAT AS
NECESSARY

For Annette, only one cathartic application of emotional connection was necessary to free her lifelong dream. Sometimes that's all you need. Most of us, however, require considerable repetition for our brain retraining to really take. I can't emphasize this enough. Otherwise, if you weather your own storm just once or twice and then don't experience the desired results, you may give up just shy of a breakthrough.

Then again, almost everyone does experience positive results immediately. First, there's the incredible relief in knowing that you can, indeed, weather the storm and survive intact. Next, there's the invigorating ease that comes with expansion. This ease is the internal correlate to the crisp freshness that follows an actual rainstorm. Frequently, until you reach that state, it's not clear how contracted you've been all along. Suddenly you're smiling more, breathing deeper, and noticing a bounce in your step. Reenergized, you now feel your dream more fully and visualize it more brilliantly. Or an infusion of creativity helps you revise and refresh your original desire to fashion a new dream that fits who you are in *this* moment of your life.

You may wonder, in light of such initial benefits, why the complete impact of this process usually requires additional storms. In certain cases, this is because a single goal links to two or more resisted emotions. When we repeat as necessary, the worst-case scenarios and resulting emotions change. Until we make it through them all, significant contraction will still exist.

PRACTICAL TIP

Sometimes reaching your goal requires weathering the storm of more than one resisted emotion.

In other cases, we need to keep revisiting the worst-case scenario because we're only partially weathering the storm. We connect to the contraction and/or emotion superficially or for just a short time before we shift from feeling our way through the issues involved into protracted thinking about them. Our mental explorations in these moments may be fascinating, maddening, or both. Yet in every variety they remain a diversion. They yank us out of the 2 X 2 process and, for the time being, keep it from reaching completion.

Then there are those pesky, recurrent disconnections, like my procrastination before writing. I think of them as ingrained human habits that will be with us for all time. The contractions and emotions they elicit, though comparatively small, come back again and again no matter how many storms we weather. That's just the way it is. Resisting this inevitability only makes the disconnections worse. Applying the 2 X 2 process, by contrast, softens their impact and shortens their duration. We quickly reconnect and free ourselves to pursue both the immediate tasks at hand and the larger dreams they serve.

The final reason to repeat as necessary, and by far the most important, is that often in weathering the storm we tap a reservoir of long-harbored and unfelt emotion, involving some of our most painful life experiences. The emotions that arise, therefore, are less about the present than the past. Each 2 X 2 process we apply is an opportunity to let both past and present emotions release, but the degree of backlog can affect how many applications are required.

In the next section, we'll explore numerous examples in which a current emotional squall connects to a much bigger tempest from the past. For now, though, it may help to have a little more perspective on how and why emotional backlogs get created in the first place. To accomplish this, let's look one last time at Annette.

Annette's unwillingness to connect to the feeling of humiliation, as discussed, only served to backfire. The longer she refused to feel it, the more stuck she grew in pursuing her dream. This, in turn, was more and more humiliating. What the story illuminates is a fundamental chink in contraction's armor. Early on, when encountering a threatening emotion, the primitive brain says, "No. Not that. Never again." But it doesn't have the ability to prevent an emotion or to block it from our experience *before* it happens. Therefore, every time Annette unintentionally landed back in a humiliating moment, she got another little precontraction taste. While the previous unfelt humiliation from her childhood was steadily intensifying over time, it was also joined periodically by this freshly stimulated humiliation. Truly, there was no *un*-humiliating place left for her to turn.

Contraction, then, is like a one-way door. New flashes of a perennially resisted emotion keep getting in, but none of it, past or present, can get out. Therefore, when at last we're ready to weather this type of storm, it usually packs a fiercer and longer wallop.

That's why backlogged emotions require so much more patience and cradling. Midstorm, they may seem overwhelming, never ending. Indeed, this is the point where many people jump ship. It often calls forth such refrains as, *Why do I have to keep dredging up the past?! Why can't I just start fresh and move forward?* The answer to this question, I hope, is now clear. All that resisted emotion from the past is still right here, right now inside us until we allow it to release. The 2 X 2 process doesn't force us back into the past but rather liberates us from it. There's no need to dwell upon who did what to whom, or when, or for how long. There's no room for done-me-wrong or woe-is-me. All of our attention is simply taken up with surfing our emotions, patiently yet quickly, toward an expansive shore.

The good news is that even the most backlogged emotions are always finite. Just like any emotion, they do bring us to that shore. They release and move on, usually far faster than we originally imagined. And this release doesn't just help the healing of old wounds—it *is* the healing. We come to find, in a poignant symmetry, that healing our past and empowering our dreams happen in the exact same way and time.

CORE CONCEPT

Backlogged emotions are always finite. Though
born in the past, they're still alive in the present.
Connecting to them is what heals our deepest
wounds *and* empowers our dreams.

Experiencing this symmetry personally, however, is a lot different than reading about it. Just last week, for instance, I met with twenty-nine-year-old Zora, who understood the process conceptually but couldn't yet feel her way through it.

Zora began our session by describing her block: "I know I'm meant to be a top-tier executive at my company," she said, "but I just can't put myself out there." Next Zora reviewed her previous efforts. She'd found the flinch—an inability to turn in the registration form for a company-sponsored leadership seminar. She'd cut to the chase—her worst-case scenario was not having anything valuable to contribute, and the feeling it induced was irrelevance. She'd attempted to weather a storm of irrelevance on three separate occasions, but wasn't able to persist for more than a few seconds without reverting back to contraction.

The missing piece, for Zora, was cradling. Stoic by nature, uneasy with vulnerability, she needed lots of encouragement to regard her feeling of irrelevance with real tenderness. Once she did, the storm was free to surge. Zora felt irrelevance mostly as a hurt in the heart and pressure in the neck. After cradling it consistently for about five minutes, she experienced, in her words, "a giant, full-body exhale." The whole thing, she told me, wasn't even very traumatic. Later that day Zora completed the registration form and sent it in, impressed at the speed of her breakthrough and confident that she'd be able to repeat when necessary.

Having finished the previous four chapters, with their extensive walk-through, you might be a little like Zora. Perhaps you grasp the big picture, but one or more of the details haven't quite clicked. That's why, before delving into part 4, it's a good idea to put down the book and get some practice.

USING EMOTIONAL CONNECTION TO GET UNSTUCK

Find the Flinch

Identify the aspect of moving forward with your vision that causes you to pull up short.

Cut to the Chase

Discover your worst-case scenario in moving forward, and determine how that outcome would make you feel.

Weather the Storm

Use all your creative power to imagine that outcome as a reality, then surf the whole cascade of emotions that comes with it.

Repeat as Necessary

Apply the above course of action whenever you get stuck again in pursuit of your goal, regarding both the same emotions and any possible new ones.

FIGURE 7

Begin working with the above formula by attempting to describe it to another person. Explaining it all in your own words helps deepen your comprehension, and it also points out those areas where you may still be a little fuzzy. Once those areas are cleared up, move on to a trial run, working with a small, manageable situation for which seeking emotional breakthrough is relatively risk free.

You might be procrastinating on a small task or project, for example. Or perhaps there's a relatively insignificant but unpleasant discussion that you haven't been able to initiate. Such cases give you the opportunity to weather a minor storm, which in turn increases your ability to stay connected during major storms. In addition this grows your trust in the process and allows you to experience tangible benefits right from the start.

The main benefit, of course, is an ability to move beyond your small chosen block. If that happens, then you're ready to tackle a bigger challenge. If it doesn't, then either repeat as necessary with the same issue, or try a couple of different issues of similar scale to help get things moving. If you're still not expanding and breaking through, pause to review the special techniques for frozen feelings in chapter 4.

PRACTICAL TIP

**When working with significant resistance,
allow yourself a period of ramp-up before
beginning the process, and a period of ramp-down
once you've completed it.**

When you're ready to work with your more significant resistance, make sure to allow enough time and privacy for the process to run its natural course. This usually involves a period of ramp-up, during which you haven't actually begun to find the flinch but are shifting into the right frame of mind to do so. It also includes a period of ramp-down, during which you let the whole experience register and settle before returning to ordinary activities.

Even the most skillful emotional connectors, however, periodically benefit from teaming up with like-minded peers. The right partners in moving through emotional resistance are people you know and trust and who support you in breaking free. The best way to use such partners is to have them listen, witness, and reflect back your experience as the process unfolds. If you get seriously lost along the way, solicit gentle, open-ended questions from your partners rather than their opinions. As a general rule, questions induce emotional connection while opinions hinder it.

It's also crucial that you choose partners who are able to "hold a space" for the emotions you're accessing. If they can't experience their own anger, for instance, they might not be able to foster a safe environment for yours. Inadvertently, such well-meaning but inappropriate partners might end up making your experience *more* difficult.

To make every one of your efforts as easy as possible, there's one more tip to keep in mind. No matter how badly you can taste success, whether about the steps along the way or your ultimate destination, try not to focus prematurely on outcomes. Whenever you push for expansion, it pulls away. Whenever you grow impatient for storms to pass, they tarry longer. Whenever you seek results from the outside world before fully opening to your internal experience, you'll be stymied in both realms.

What's holding you back, to be sure, can only be found in one place—the present moment. That's exactly where breakthroughs happen as well. As you become more and more able to cultivate emotional connection in the present moment, without imposing any schedules or demands, the future begins to take care of itself.

PART FOUR

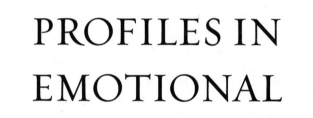

PROFILES IN EMOTIONAL CONNECTION

ADDICTION AND COMPULSION

OVER THE NEXT THREE CHAPTERS you'll meet a wide variety of people who broke through significant, real-life blocks using the very same techniques we've just covered. Every profile presented contains one or more key refinements to those techniques. The key refinements are introduced first within the profiles themselves and then further explored under their own headings. Each one will help you maximize your own effectiveness with emotional connection even if the profile with which it appears doesn't seem pertinent to your specific issues.

With that in mind, let's turn our attention to addiction and compulsion. The definitions of these two terms are almost as varied and confusing as the ones for emotion. Here's a rough synthesis: addiction is a persistent, uncontrollable action that is known to be harmful; compulsion is a repetitive urge to perform an action for irrational or unconscious reasons. While most of us don't suffer from full-blown addictions (unless you count coffee and sugar), we're all prone to compulsions of one kind or another. They show up mostly in our relation to food, sex, entertainment, and stress relief. Compulsions are sometimes referred to as soft addictions, highlighting the way these two phenomena are similar, related, and to varying degrees destructive.

In counseling hundreds of people about their addictions and compulsions, I've come to my own description that encompasses them both: the continuous use of any substance or activity to create disconnection from one's emotions. Let me put that another way: with the practice of emotional connection, virtually all addictions and compulsions cease. That doesn't mean people never use the substance or partake in the activity again. Instead, it means they become able to choose if, when, and how to do so with complete conscious awareness. They go from being irresponsible to responsible, from powerless to powerful.

At first this may seem like a controversial claim. Isn't addiction a disease? Isn't the first step in every Twelve Step program to admit that we're completely powerless over our addiction? The answer to both questions is yes. But the root condition underlying the disease is emotional disconnection, and we're only powerless as long as we remain in that condition.

CORE CONCEPT

**Addictions and compulsions are strategies
for emotional disconnection. They lose the
majority of their power once consistent
emotional connection is established.**

As with all the principles and practices in this book, I hope that rather than taking my word for this, you experiment in the laboratory of your own life. Of course this isn't medical advice, and if you're in a treatment program for addiction, please proceed only with the consent and guidance of your doctor or sponsor.* In fact, whether your own

---

*When discussing how to work with addiction in this chapter, I don't deal directly with the hardcore physical withdrawal symptoms caused by many substances. The same principles and practices do apply to those symptoms, however, even if and when they require additional medical intervention.

coping mechanism includes addiction, compulsion, or both, I recommend beginning your experimentation in a very gradual manner. If you tend toward compulsive gambling, for example, don't set out to quit cold turkey via emotional connection or even to skip a single planned trip to the casino. Instead, make your initial goal simply to notice a little more than usual what's going on in your body before, during, and after the trip. Then, after a few such experiments with heightened awareness, assess whether it's time to add one of the key refinements suggested in this chapter.

What you'll find along the way is that addiction and compulsion play a central role in the battle between emotions that need to be felt and contractions that are designed to keep that from happening. When a contraction can't do its work all alone, it calls in addiction and/or compulsion as reinforcements. They're a central part of the primitive brain's arsenal for keeping us "safe" from unwanted emotions, and they operate by creating a temporary but potent protective effect. They protect us specifically from the *emotional* reality of any moment. Unfortunately, this effect grows less successful over time, while the personal fallout continues to mount.

I'm beginning this profiles section on the subject of addiction and compulsion for two reasons. First, addictive and compulsive behaviors play an ever-increasing role in our society. There's not a single one of us who isn't seriously impacted by them at one point or another. Second, these behaviors present some of the greatest challenges to emotional connection. Therefore, fine-tuning our skills in this arena will make everything else seem a whole lot easier.

Before we begin, I invite you to reflect for a few moments on your own repertoire of addictions and compulsions. What substances and behaviors have traditionally soothed, numbed, or distracted you during times of stress and emotional upset? The list of possibilities is nearly endless, because almost anything can be used to serve those functions, even seemingly healthy activities like exercise and meditation. To zero in on your own list, just think about what you do, or long to do, when things become too much. Think about what you turn to when facing a responsibility that you'd rather avoid. Think about what you get sucked into when you're well aware that you should be doing something else. Once you've completed the list, read the profiles below with a keen eye toward applying each of their refinements to your own situation.

The Issue: Compulsive Overeating

Nancy S.—Family Practice Physician, 45, Melbourne, Florida

Nancy had overcome a great deal of adversity in her life to achieve a high degree of success. Her practice was overflowing with patients, yet she also had a full, competent staff to keep the responsibilities and stress level manageable. Her marriage of fifteen years was flourishing, and her two kids were thriving on all fronts. Nancy attributed much of this bounty to the personal introspection she'd done following a first marriage that began in medical school and ended in her residency. During that introspection she discovered the childhood wounds that were unconsciously at play in her choices and behaviors, and she took a yearlong leave from the fast track in order for real healing to take place.

Even with all that healing, however, and the nearly two decades of blessings that followed, Nancy still suffered from a lifelong struggle with obesity. She yo-yoed between fifty and seventy pounds above her goal weight and always felt uncomfortable, lethargic, and imprisoned within her own body. No amount of dieting, exercise, prayer, or self-talk seemed to make a difference. Growing more and more desperate through the years, Nancy became willing to try things that as a doctor she knew full well were snake oil, just to make sure there was no stone left unturned in her search for a lasting solution.

Nancy had a gentle manner and a sharp intellect. Together, Nancy and I undertook a mission to understand her relationship with food from the inside out. We began by looking at a typical situation in which Nancy's eating habits were out of alignment with both her desire for weight loss and her actual appetite. She described flopping on the couch after a long day at work and with the kids finally in bed. Sometimes she'd turn on the TV, and at other times she'd curl up with a book. Either way, a thought bubble would soon appear, containing an image of whatever ice-cream container was currently in the freezer. The more she pushed the image away, the more insistently it would reappear. In the end it would always win, and soon Nancy would be off the couch and in the kitchen, spooning out the ice cream into an oversized bowl. This whole sequence of events would transpire with Nancy in a kind of hypnotic trance. The trance would continue as she returned to the couch and hurriedly emptied the bowl. Afterward she'd feel bloated, guilty, vowing to break this pattern once and for all, starting tomorrow.

Sound familiar? Of course that particular tomorrow never really came. The closest Nancy got to it was a workshop she took on "mindful eating." There, she discovered that most of the time her desserts weren't even enjoyable. She'd take bite after bite on automatic pilot, barely tasting their flavor while reabsorbing herself in the night's book or TV. At the workshop she learned to pay attention to the whole eating process and to savor each spoonful of her chosen treat slowly and fully. This is a great practice, and at first it worked. Nancy was able to cut her dessert consumption in half for a few months, but then little by little she fell back into her old, distracted ways.

Once Nancy was versed in the 2 X 2 process, I asked her to walk through the entire dessert experience in her mind's eye. The first thing she noticed was that along with the ice-cream thought bubble came a physical contraction just beneath her diaphragm. It felt, she said, like a baby reaching adamantly for some bauble. I asked her, if the baby could speak, what it would say. "Gimme that!" she replied, repeating it over and over.

This, alas, is the nature of compulsive desire. It's a relentless one-note assault that seemingly won't let up until we give in. I asked Nancy not to fight it but to stay connected with it as the scenario continued to unfold. Next, she saw herself getting up and hurrying to the freezer. I suggested that she shift into slow motion, seeing what else the 2 X 2 process might help her uncover. On the way to the freezer the contraction persisted, and along with it came the expectation of approaching fulfillment. She could practically taste this sensation, and in fact her mouth began to water. At the freezer door I asked her to pause, to be with those sensations for a few moments more. Now the contraction eased, and the expectation grew to a powerful excitement that rose in waves through her whole trunk. I invited Nancy to get microscopic with the waves. She shut her eyes and concentrated silently for a moment. Then she told me it was like a little girl, maybe five years old, jumping up and down inside her.

I then suggested that Nancy kneel beside the imaginary girl, that she watch carefully as the girl continued to jump up and down, and that she also stay connected to the physical sensations inside. After a few moments I wondered aloud why this little girl was so happy. At first, reflexively, Nancy responded that the girl just loved ice cream and couldn't wait to get inside that freezer.

I instructed Nancy to open the freezer door and take out the ice cream, but still in slow motion and without losing touch with the girl or her own inner sensations. She did so and went on to remove the ice cream, take off the lid, and grab a spoon from the dish rack. But then she paused, broke free of the vision, opened her eyes, and looked at me with surprise.

"It's not the ice cream that she wants so badly," Nancy proclaimed. "It's the attention. I mean, maybe this is just psychobabble, but it feels like she's the playful part of me and the only time I ever let her out, or even acknowledge her, is with sweets." I pointed out that a little judging was seeping into her attention, and that it would be good to acknowledge that without resistance and then continue to provide the little girl with the attention she craved.

Nancy soon teared up. "Oh my God," she moaned. "Now all the playfulness is gone, and there's just sadness. Ick. This is what I've fought my whole life. I'm so tired of it. Do we have to go there? Again? After the divorce it practically took up my whole therapy." More judging, I noted, and asked Nancy, if possible, to stay with the sadness a bit longer. She did, which led to a minute or so of muffled sobbing. Then Nancy settled into a calming expansion.

"I really do know all about this," she told me. "I've been over the story a million times." She started to tell it once more, for my benefit, but I intervened. The story's not so important, I assured her. I had no doubt that she'd relived and analyzed it to death. All that mattered now was what she'd just experienced.

She crumpled up her tissue, puzzled. "What do you mean?"

I suggested she tune back in to her body and see for herself. "Well," she said, "I do feel better. Sort of like . . . more at home."

As our session went on, Nancy and I discussed the way that the deep sadness of her childhood was, for so many years, too much to bear. So her system contracted around it and kept her safe. But in order for that to work, since the sadness was so powerful, Nancy had to compulsively overeat. The appearance of her "Gimme that!" contraction whenever it appeared was a reliable indication that an emotion, most likely sadness, had arisen to be felt. To feel it, though painful at times, was ultimately more satisfying than the ice cream. Perhaps just as important at this point in her life was the recognition that dealing with the sadness by feeling it wouldn't lead to any extra pounds. In fact, it was the very thing that would allow the pounds to come off.

Over time as the pounds did come off—and stay off—Nancy also experienced other benefits. The more sadness she felt, the less intensely she was gripped by her compulsion. The reason her compulsion diminished was because less and less of the old sadness remained. Once truly felt, it dissipated. Plus, her system got the message that sadness wasn't actually dangerous. So not only did the compulsion ease, but the contraction that gave rise to it eased as well.

Key Refinements

THE RECONSTRUCTED WALK-THROUGH

You might notice that I didn't ask Nancy to find the flinch, cut to the chase, and weather the storm. That's because compulsions often require a variation on the basic formula. Nancy's compulsion qualified due to years of giving in to it that had made the underlying emotion harder than usual to access. I sensed this was true from the outset of our work together, especially because Nancy had already done so much introspection and had not yet reached a sufficient level of healing from this core wound.

Stubborn compulsions also involve subtle dimensions. Reconstructing the usual compulsive scenario almost always reveals those dimensions, as long as the walk-through is slow enough to let exquisite attention be paid to every inner detail. In Nancy's case, proceeding any quicker would likely have caused us to stop at the excited little girl and miss the essential sad one underneath.

IMAGES AND PERSONAS

Many people, like Nancy, are skeptical of pop psychology concepts like the "inner child." And well they should be, since no such thing really exists. Such imaginary constructions are helpful for some people and get in the way for others. With emotional connection, on the other hand, something similar yet far more natural occurs for almost everyone. We sense emotions not just with inner feeling but also with images.

PRACTICAL TIP

Sometimes you may sense emotions not just with inner feeling but also with images.

If we connect to anger roiling in our stomach, for instance, we might also *see* that anger. It might show up as a mental image of fire or a molten cauldron, or perhaps as morphing shapes or just a static red ball. Noting such images and letting them be part of the overall emotional experience is a great help in creating connection and flow.

When we're willing to include these images, they often transform into images of ourselves, and particularly of ourselves as children. It's during childhood that we felt our emotions with the most power and least filtering. It's also during childhood that we experienced many of the hardships and hurts that came to shape our characters. No wonder, then, that these images of our young selves arise during emotional connection and with greatest intensity when our most vulnerable feelings are afoot.

On a personal note, whenever I feel raw and small, stung with life's inevitable disappointments, the emotions always come with the exact same image of myself. I'm five years old, swinging around my mailbox, gazing with frustration and heartbreak at the chaotic home from which I just fled. I don't know whether that image of my mailbox swinging ever really happened, and it doesn't matter. As long as I cradle the image, along with its corresponding sensations, it brings me to expansion as quickly and peacefully as possible.

Like Nancy and me, you'll make great strides in releasing emotional resistance by embracing these childhood images whenever they appear. If you feel self-conscious doing so, embrace that too. And keep an eye out as well for any inner sounds, tastes, and textures. They frequently emerge also at vital moments from what psychologists call the *imaginal realm* and can be wonderful aids in deepening your emotional presence.

The Issue: Alcoholism and Smoking

Alan K.—Forest Ranger, 38, White Mountain, Maine

Alan first developed a drinking habit in his college fraternity, but it later took greater hold when he was stationed for lengthy stretches in remote forest lookouts. Those assignments were long past, but the addiction had still remained and threatened his marriage and family. With a strong desire to quit, Alan had been through two stays at a residential treatment facility and was in both AA and a hospital support group. This was keeping the drinking under control, but now, as is common, Alan had developed a compensatory smoking problem, essentially trading one addiction for another.

Upon meeting Alan, I immediately liked his wry, been-there-done-it-all manner. I told him that I didn't care whether he stopped smoking or not. That was his choice, and my job was simply to support him in the discovery of what created the need to smoke in the first place. As you'll see, this complete acceptance and valuing of Alan as a person, with or without his addiction, helped create the necessary climate for our work together. Alan told me he appreciated this candor and that he was "sick to death" of furrowed brows and veiled judgments, most of all his own. Above everything, he felt tired, wrung out, and bitter from a destructive force that seemed to dwarf even his "higher power." I attempted to normalize these feelings, reminding Alan that even the best treatment programs have a very low success rate.

I asked Alan to tell me how the decision to have each cigarette occurred for him. After thinking about it for a while, he described a nearly universal experience related to all varieties of addiction. First a switch went off in his mind, alerting him that it was time to partake. After that, it was a done deal, whether he actually partook right away or hours later and also whether the current craving seemed more physical or emotional. This switch, I explained to Alan, flips specifically to avoid our worst-case scenario, which is about an internal experience rather than an external event. In other words, here the worst-case scenario and the feelings connected to it are one and the same. But because addiction is so overpowering, without some special techniques it's impossible to find out what those feelings really are.

Would it be possible, I wondered, for Alan to create a small space between the switch going off and the decision being made? What if he got the internal message *You're going to have a cigarette*, and his response was, "Okay, maybe, but let's put off the final decision for a little bit." Alan wanted to know how long I had in mind, and I suggested one minute. I went on to clarify that the time period was less important than what went on within it. And for that, no surprise, I suggested the 2 X 2 process. I invited Alan to pay very close attention to all the feelings and sensations that arose when he practiced what I call "done-deal delay." If he did so, one possibility was that the decision to have the cigarette would change. Another possibility was that the decision would still stand. If that happened, I told him, go for it. Smoke away.

Alan liked the freedom in that and vowed to try it a number of times during the next week. When he returned for another session, the report was mixed. Most of the time he made it through the whole minute and then went on to have the smoke. About a fifth of the time, he made it through the minute, and the desire to smoke decreased, always coming back full-strength eventually but often not for quite a while. The rest of the time, Alan got frustrated, overcome by the sensations, and opted for the smoke even before the minute was over.

From my perspective this was all great news. I explained to Alan that he was allowing himself to have a brand-new experience—totally the opposite of his usual attempts at will power. With willpower, one part of us fights against another, such as the part that wants to quit smoking doing battle against the part that doesn't. This can work for a time, but almost always with a subsequent pushback in which the defeated part of us finds a way to get expressed. A pushback, such as Alan's trade of alcohol for cigarettes, tends to have negative consequences and thwart our good intentions. Another example of the pushback is the dry drunk, someone who gives up the physical dependency on alcohol but holds on to the overall addictive behavior.

In the absence of such self-opposition, a dynamic, moment-by-moment self-acceptance can take root. We can then use the 2 X 2 process to experience ourselves fully and to make decisions that are peacefully sustainable, because no parts get banished, and therefore no pushback is necessary. I suggested that Alan continue to familiarize himself with self-acceptance, adding more and more time to his done-deal delay whenever possible, as long as no strain was involved. In addition to the principle of self-acceptance, I introduced Alan to what I call the "no fail zone," which is crucial for handling those moments when 2 X 2-ing our sensations becomes overwhelming and we just can't continue.

This is how the no-fail zone works. We look at each instance in which self-acceptance has fallen short and we've gone on to indulge not as a problem but instead as an opportunity. In all such instances an emotion appears that is especially challenging for us to feel. Provided with this information, we're now alert and prepared for the next time it shows up. When it does, we take special care to go slower and get more microscopic. We learn to pinpoint this particular emotion, opening to it in smaller, less lengthy amounts. The more we do so, the better we become at it. Our persistence, in turn, draws down the emotion's intensity.

The next week, Alan returned for his appointment with great excitement. He was finding, to his surprise, that he could often keep the 2 X 2 process going between the switch and the done deal for not just minutes but hours. He didn't require special time for this, apart from his other life activities, but rather could keep checking in and surfing the emotional waves right alongside daily life. He still smoked, but much less, and the pull of the cigarettes was diminishing significantly.

Inspired by these developments, I asked Alan for an update on his experience in the no-fail zone. He told me that what usually tripped him up was a sense of panic. This panic arose as an insistent command: *Can't be here. Gotta get away. Gotta run.* When he got slower and more microscopic, the panic projected internal images of Alan as a child, cowering in the bathroom as his alcoholic father rampaged through the house. Alan was starting to see that while his father never actually hurt him, the legacy of this fear had lingered for years. Feeling this emotion fully after so long wasn't easy, and all he could currently take was about five seconds at a time. Those five seconds had the power to be life changing, I promised Alan, and they would increase exponentially if he kept at it.

Alan did keep at it. At the time of this writing he's been nearly smoke free for three years. On the few occasions that he has smoked, it didn't lead to hitting bottom or anything similar. Within a day or two, he was able to employ the no-fail zone to learn what was really happening. These times brought Alan into contact not just with the fear, but also with another buried emotion: anger. He met this anger with the advanced techniques for feeling described in chapter 4, especially breathing into it and applying posture-movement-sound. It left him raw but also more alive and less reactive. In addition, his wife and kids came to see a huge difference in his everyday demeanor. He grew softer, much more approachable. His newfound self-acceptance, to their relief and delight, was leading him to greater acceptance of them as well.

Key Refinements

DONE-DEAL DELAY

The storms that arise from staving off an addictive or compulsive response can be uniquely difficult to weather. That's why they're best approached incrementally, starting with just a minute or less, and then gradually adding more time for 2 X 2 at whatever rate and amount fit you best.

When incorporating done-deal delay, any duration of storm weathering is positive, even if it's immediately followed by your usual, numbing indulgence. Mere seconds of delay still provide tangible proof that you *can* tolerate the sensations that come from declining to indulge. This strengthens your muscle of connection, as well as your motivation to keep working it. Done-deal delay, as you can gather, is a less punishing alternative to cold turkey.

SELF-ACCEPTANCE

Most of the time, we're at mental war with ourselves. That's because one part of our minds is telling another part what to do. That other part doesn't like to be ordered around and usually won't obey for very long. Plus, it has its own contradictory view to promote and is just as pushy about it. In a mind that's at all shut down, there's only enough room for one victor at any given time. So the war drags on between these two opposing parts, with one constantly pushing back against the other in an endless cycle of either/or.

When expansion takes hold, however, suddenly there's enough room for two points of view. They can exist side by side, beheld in our more open minds as equally valid. They can even become allies in a course of action that takes each perspective into full account. In the synthesis that results, brand-new possibilities often emerge, ones that could never have been discovered as long as the war continued to rage. Such an expanded consciousness is often referred to as both/and. Describing it, the great twentieth-century writer F. Scott Fitzgerald remarked that, "The test of a first-rate intelligence is the ability to hold two opposing ideas in mind at the same time and still function." When viewed through the lens of emotional connection, we see that this attribute allows a mind not only to function but to perform at its peak.

CORE CONCEPT

Willpower never works in the long run, but self-acceptance almost always does.

Willpower is an either/or proposition. In Alan's case, it first appeared when the authoritarian part of his mind tried to reign in his indulgent side. *Stop drinking now!* it commanded. *Okay, you're right, I'm sorry,* the indulgent side replied, temporarily pretending to submit. *But now it's time to start smoking,* it soon decreed, *and there's not a damn thing you can do about it!* From that point on, it was back and forth incessantly between reproach and release, sometimes over the course of a month and other times within a mere minute. And Alan didn't just side with whatever part of him was currently on top—he actually fused with it.

Self-acceptance is a both/and proposition. As Alan became more familiar with it, he was able to referee his internal dialogue rather than get whipsawed by it. The result went something like this: *You want me to smoke. I hear you and understand why. And you want me to quit forever, which I also totally get. No one's wrong here. Let's not fight. Instead, would it be alright if we experiment with another option?* During the truce that followed, there was plenty of time and

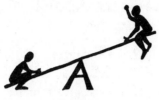

Either/Or

One desire or view always dominates, but only temporarily.

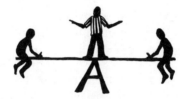

Both/And

*No winners or losers. An internal referee helps
keep the peace and explore alternatives.*

FIGURE 8

space for Alan to deepen his 2 X 2 practice. This, in turn, allowed him
to quit smoking with no pushback.

Most of the world's cultures have relied upon a strict moral code to
keep people and their messy impulses in place. For the most part, we
still live on a "Thou shalt not" planet. We also, as a result, see signs of
furious pushback in every direction. Even though self-acceptance is
a peaceful and effective alternative to this eternal either/or battle, it
doesn't get much press. That's because, to many people, a both/and
orientation seems like "anything goes." They think that it's a license
to act out our worst impulses and desires. After all, didn't I tell Alan
it was okay if he smoked?

It's true, I did, and what I meant was that I wouldn't judge Alan no
matter what happened. It was that freedom from judgment that
allowed him to truly pay attention to his impulses for the first time,
rather than just indulge or condemn them. This kind of attention,

when coupled with emotional connection, allowed him to embody his morals from the inside out.

But what does all this talk about morals and culture have to do with you and your own addictions and compulsions? The answer is that you, along with the most significant people in your life, have likely internalized some aspects of the cultural bias against self-acceptance. This bias will probably emerge when you set out to greet your destructive behaviors as a mentally detached referee (both/and) instead of getting lost in the fight (either/or). At times it might seem wrong, bad, or even sinful to explore these unwanted aspects of yourself with compassionate curiosity.

If this happens, you can catch it quickly by noting the pinched, stern sensation it produces in your body. Standing in judgment, it turns out, almost never feels positive or peaceful. But using the 2 X 2 process to explore exactly how it does feel, physically, restores the expansive inner state necessary for self-acceptance to flourish. So whenever your mind becomes a hostile environment, don't seek to change it. Instead, let your body do all the work.

Choosing this body-centered approach has one more important benefit. Without it, self-acceptance can become dry, distant, and ultimately ineffective. We see ourselves clearly but as if from a mile away. We understand what's led to our addictions and compulsions but without ever really feeling any of it. In this case we gain knowledge without wisdom and therefore don't really change much at all. Alan was in danger of just such a fate. He'd learned so much about himself through recovery but hadn't yet experienced the healing that comes from direct emotional connection. Once he did experience that healing, all his hard-won understanding could finally lead to real-world transformation.

THE NO-FAIL ZONE

As you can recognize from Alan's experience, the no-fail zone is often the only thing that allows us to keep going when previously we've been discouraged and deterred. It's a frame of reference that's helpful with addiction, compulsion, and any other attempt at emotional connection. Every single time we're unable to remain in connection, despite our best efforts, can be seen as an invitation to cradle the sense of failure directly but without buying into its verdict.

PRACTICAL TIP

Feeling the raw sensation of failure in your body, when necessary, doesn't mean you must *believe* that you've actually failed.

Next, once expanded, we revisit the experience to find out what, specifically, undermined our efforts. Was it analyzing, judging, assessing, or bargaining? Was it distraction? An especially intense contraction? The strength of the emotion itself? This vital information, obtainable no other way, turns our previous disconnection into a bona fide victory. Then, when next facing the same thorny experience, we're alerted to the need for pinpointing.

PINPOINTING

To pinpoint an emotion requires that we take the process ever more incrementally, just as with done-deal delay, until there's no need to disconnect. This is akin to any project that's overwhelming in its entirety but grows manageable once we break it down into the smallest possible parts and tackle them one at a time.

Panic, to stay with Alan's example, is often unbearable when taken as one giant storm. But when pinpointed, it might crystallize into a series of images or become sweaty palms, shallow breathing, or a racing heart. If focused on with gentle precision, these discrete occurrences are usually tolerable enough for a brief time. Over a longer period of time such occurrences add up, and frequently we find ourselves all the way through the storm. Pinpointing may occur many times in one long session of 2 X 2, during which we stop and start as necessary to avoid taking on too much. Or, it may occur over a series of sessions in which we return to the same storm repeatedly.

The Issue: Compulsive Sexuality

Randall B.—Bank Executive, 51, Seattle, Washington

Randall had a commanding presence, deep voice, and movie-star good looks. At first, he was more concerned with confidentiality than emotional connection. In line for the CFO position of a Fortune 500 company, he had a lot riding on it. Plus, he was about to tell me things that even his wife didn't know. I carefully reviewed the details of our confidentiality agreement with him before diving in, and then when reasonably comfortable, Randall gave it to me straight.

"Listen," he said, "I know full well what this is all about, but I just can't seem to stop myself." He went on to describe a series of sexual encounters with men, although he definitely didn't consider himself gay or even bisexual. Each encounter happened in the same way: first a round of e-mails through Craigslist, then text messaging, then a brief encounter at a hotel or adult bookstore. Throughout the lead-up to the experience, until its eventual completion, Randall felt a steadily growing surge of adrenaline. It made him feel incredibly awake, alert, and alive. Then, after the encounter was over, Randall would feel deeply ashamed and despondent. This cycle began a few years previous to our meeting, when Randall's career star first began to rise, and now that he was heading for the stratosphere, it was increasing in frequency every month.

Randall also described what he considered the source of his compulsion—two years of sexual molestation at the hands of a popular high-school track coach. He'd buried the experience successfully until his first son was born. At that point, scared of what it all meant, he finally shared it with his church pastor. The counseling that followed brought him a sense of clarity and peace, which remained until this new round of compulsive activity.

Hearing all this, I honored Randall for having the courage to share it years ago with his pastor and now also with me. I told him that while some important healing had obviously taken place during his previous counseling, a part of him was still acting out for attention. I explained the way emotions create destructive patterns until fully felt, an idea we've touched on earlier, especially regarding Annette. I invoked the incisive words of the twentieth-century English writer Kenneth Tynan, who said, "We seek the teeth to match our wounds." Tynan's quote helps us see the way many destructive emotional patterns are linked to people. Until we fully embrace and heal a damaging experience, we're often condemned to find people who restimulate that earlier pain. Once our healing happens, however, there's nowhere for those "teeth" to go.

But all that was just more information, background really, and Randall was desperate to regain control. I gave him a crash course in the 2 X 2 process, and we got to work. That work entailed a reconstructed walkthrough of his last compulsive sexual encounter. We attempted to stay slow and micro all the way through the posting of an ad on Craigslist to the encounter itself. We needed to do this numerous times, stopping and starting, invoking the no-fail zone often, partly because the issue was so delicate and partly because Randall's personality—type À and defensive—made adequate emotional connection more difficult than usual.

Our breakthrough occurred as Randall saw himself outside a motel room, about to knock, knowing that his sexual liaison was waiting on the other side of the door. The adrenaline rush was tremendous. Even though the scenario was merely memory, Randall felt like his heart was jumping out of his chest. His breath was fast and shallow, and his forehead began to perspire. I asked Randall to get even slower than before, to let his attention sink into the very center of the rush.

As he did, suddenly there was no rush. In its place was a miserable trembling. Now Randall saw himself not as an adult, but as the teenage boy who was, yet again, about to be molested. The predominant feeling was one of utter powerlessness. Randall felt powerless to resist the influential and respected authority figure who faced him, powerless to resist the experience's undeniable physical pleasure, and powerless to resist his guilt and shame for not trying to escape. Gently, I guided Randall to sink his attention into the center of this powerlessness, just as he had done with the rush. This extreme state of vulnerability felt both threatening and overwhelming.

To his great credit, Randall stayed with the powerlessness till it began to flow and release and until his breath softened into a long, expansive sigh. After about a minute I brought Randall's mind back to the motel-room door. I asked him to assess his next move from this current state. He said he wanted to leave the motel, be by himself, perhaps go for a drive, and spend some time at a nearby lake. Mindful of a possible pushback, I asked if there was any part of him that wanted to enter the motel room. He said yes, but that it was a small part and without a strong inclination. I encouraged him to let that part of himself be present, too (both/and), there in the office and then also later on. He nodded in agreement.

Over the next three months, Randall called me twice. Each time the compulsion had returned with more strength than he expected. The first time, in response, we did the same walk-through as before, only now projecting it into the future (a variation of the worst-case scenario), imagining slowly and in micro what would happen if he went through with the prospective encounter. At the end of the imagined scene, Randall felt a shudder of shame so powerful that he nearly went into shock. Courageously, however, he managed to stay with it and in the process facilitated a final piece of his healing. This healing acted as a compulsion eraser, and Randall hung up from our phone call feeling strong and clear.

The second time Randall called me, we took the opposite walkthrough, imagining slowly and in micro what would happen if he *didn't* indulge the compulsion (another variation of the worst-case scenario). This led Randall to a sense of profound letdown, complete with boredom, petulance, hopelessness, and isolation. In meeting each of these states via 2 X 2, Randall untangled another vital part of the abuse's legacy. He was literally detoxing from the adrenaline cycle with its hypnotic highs and crushing lows, feeling his way toward a more even-keeled existence. I counseled Randall that it would likely take some time for him to find real solace and the more subtly pleasant dimensions in such a rush-free life. While he took a wait-and-see attitude on that front, the walk-through did defuse his need to indulge.

Following these two phone calls, Randall's desire to act out lessened markedly. There were, nonetheless, a few additional times when the compulsion reflared. During these times, instead of calling me, Randall was able to perform one or more walk-through varieties by himself and with equally successful results.

By repeating as necessary, Randall came to understand how professional success often highlights the ways we don't feel totally worthy of it. He realized that the healing provided by emotional connection was allowing him, at last, to feel completely deserving. This change eliminated the need to sabotage himself. Therefore, his compulsion and its associated rush lost even more of their lure.

The following year Randall did go on to become CFO, a position he still holds. He tells me that sometimes his urges reappear, but now they feel manageable and not so threatening. Eventually he decided to share the whole healing journey with his wife, even though he knew how challenging it would be for her. The initial results were rocky and sent them straight to couple's counseling. While their progress as a couple is another story, to date they are still together.

Key Refinement

THE ADRENALINE FACTOR

During my work with Randall, I had no preconceived or favored outcome. His own preference was to stop the sexual encounters, and therefore I wanted to help. If our exploration had led to Randall's acceptance of himself as gay or bisexual, that result would've been equally welcome.

Once we began exploring, however, it quickly became clear that Randall's work was more about emotional connection than sexual orientation. How did I know? Adrenaline was the key. Any compulsive behavior that brings about an adrenaline rush—such as gambling or shoplifting—is an indicator of major emotional repression.

PRACTICAL TIP

An adrenaline rush signals emotional repression.

The force of the rush is what splits us off from the rest of who we are and is commensurate with the wounding it represses. Without the rush, we wouldn't be able to transgress our values.

In working with compulsions that generate an adrenaline rush, experiment with the same three approaches that Randall and I employed. The first approach, applicable in the aftermath of a compulsive episode, is a reconstructed walk-through as described fully in Nancy's profile.

The second approach combines elements of the walk-through and cut to the chase. Rather than attempting to identify the worst thing that could happen from proceeding with a current compulsion, let the scenario of its future indulgence play out, uncontrolled and unedited, in your mind's eye. It's important in this variation to explore the comedown following your compulsive activity as fully as the indulging itself. That's because often, like with Randall's shudder of shame, it's in the comedown that the emotional gold lies.

The third approach is the reverse of the second and is useful not just when adrenaline is present but also with any addiction or compulsion. Here, imagine the experiential fallout from denying your urge entirely. This allows you to preview the whole sequence of reactions and emotions that deprivation will likely bring. Following the 2 X 2 process through this preview serves two purposes: (1) you derive all the usual benefits from emotional connection, and (2) if you decide to follow this conjured deprivation with the real-life version, it's bound to sting a whole lot less.

The second and third approaches both require that you're willing and able to practice done-deal delay. To help in that regard, think of the presence of adrenaline as an enormous stop sign. When you feel it, wait to indulge. Without waiting for at least a half hour, it's impossible to envision a sufficiently unhurried and detailed scenario of either indulgence or deprivation. But if you can't stop, remember not to get down on yourself. Instead, gently invoke the no-fail zone and look for what made that particular episode so overpowering. Then, try to stop again next time with the aid of this added information

Whenever you can stop, use the approaches here not only to get to the emotional underpinnings of your compulsion, but also to bring about a fully expanded state. From there, you'll be in a reliable position to evaluate your options. Remember, breaking through addiction and compulsion doesn't mean that you forswear any behavior as universally wrong or bad. Instead, no longer ruled by emotional resistance, you're free to make conscious choices about such behavior that best suit each unique circumstance. Even if your renouncing of the compulsion remains fixed and you choose to abstain continually regardless of circumstance, each "no, thank you" will be freshly reconfirmed and internally harmonious. You won't have to rely on willpower to enforce your choice and therefore won't face any pushback either.

The Issue: Compulsive Overeating

Kelly S.—*Tech Support, 29, Ames, Iowa*

I decided to begin and end this chapter with profiles about overeating because 1) it's so prevalent and 2) nearly all cases are caused by compulsion. Kelly, for instance, was 130 pounds overweight. Kelly's own body was so repugnant to her that she covered every mirror in the house able to reflect anything below the neck. As we worked together over the phone, I learned what had led her to this state. The details of that story aren't so relevant, but what happened in one particular session could model a turning point for many.

Kelly's regular MO went something like this: A painful or uncomfortable emotion would arise. She would stuff it down by eating. That initial feeling would soon disappear, but not long after, she'd be overcome by guilt and shame. Often, she'd attempt to stuff down those responses with more food, but it never seemed to work, and the weight just kept increasing.

As we continued our conversation, Kelly reported that talking about her food issues was making her agitated and that a bag of chips on the counter beckoned. I asked Kelly if she was really ready to explore a choice other than disconnection through eating, even if just for a short while. She said yes, and I invited her to proceed to the largest mirror in the house. After some foreboding and hesitation, she agreed. Once Kelly was in front of the mirror, I suggested that she put down the phone, remove the mirror's covering, and engage in the 2 X 2 process while looking at her entire body. I told her to pick up the receiver again whenever she had a need or desire to share.

One minute went by, then another. Soon five minutes passed. I fretted about my decision to stay removed from Kelly's process, wondering in what directions her thoughts and emotions were traveling. Just then, though, Kelly returned to the phone. She recounted moving through contraction to fear and back again. Following that, she weathered a powerful pang of self-revulsion. Right then, Kelly recalled, she realized that it was possible to leave the room and grab some chips without my ever knowing. Instead, though, she stayed put. Not long after her urge to bolt came wave upon wave of grief. She cradled this emotional holdover from her childhood, spontaneously whispering the words "It's alright, it's alright" over and over again. Then she was moved to cradle herself physically, putting both arms around her middle and rocking from side to side. Most of her minutes away from the phone were spent in this way. By the time she came back, the sadness remained but was now accompanied by a palpable tenderness.

After listening to Kelly's report, I asked her whether at this very moment she still wanted those chips. She said no, absolutely not, that she just wanted to curl up tightly in her duvet. We ended our session early so she could do just that. Before hanging up, however, Kelly agreed to uncover all the mirrors in her house and to meet each food compulsion during the next week with 2 X 2-ing in sight of her full reflection.

Key Refinement

STAND IN THE FIRE

This session with Kelly highlights what has been implicit in each of the preceding profiles—the need beneath every addiction and compulsion is emotional connection. Whenever these urges first strike, they bludgeon us with the idea that succumbing to our current desire will lead to ultimate fulfillment. Inevitably, while disconnected, we take the bait. Then the next time, despite having been duped over and over, we take the bait once more and repeat the futile cycle. But if we follow the 2 X 2 process long enough during any addictive or compulsive passage, the initial desire relinquishes the stage to our deeper, truer emotional need. And this need actually *can* be fulfilled.

Kelly's mirror practice was akin to standing in a fire. Taking such a risk is scary because it seems like we'll incinerate. But instead we remain standing, unharmed, and it's our destructive desire that burns away. So this refinement isn't about one specific act, like standing in front of a mirror to deal with overeating (though that might be helpful for you). What it's about is using whatever you can dream up to help facilitate and lengthen your own fire time. If you're a gambler, it might involve framing the overdraft notices from your bank. If you're a drug abuser, it might involve surrounding yourself with photos of estranged loved ones.

At first consideration this idea may seem punitive, like rubbing your nose in it, but the real objective is to break the trance that might otherwise send you fleeing from the 2 X 2 process and straight into the arms of your habit. If you feel drawn to employ such a visceral aid, experiment with whatever comes to mind until something really works. When it does, you'll find yourself fully in touch with the deeper need beneath your compulsion. Then, whether all at once or with time, you'll finally be able to meet it.

IN THE WORKPLACE

D ESPITE THE MAJOR INROADS to the business community made by champions of emotional intelligence, many top executives are still in the dark. "Feelings don't belong in the workplace"—to this day it's a common refrain, although feelings never require an invitation to show up and always cause the most trouble when they're denied or disparaged. Even in more enlightened companies, the relationship to emotions often remains rocky. This rocky relationship can lead to flawed strategy and great financial loss. Our first profile in this chapter describes how such an occurrence was narrowly avoided. It's longer and more complex than the profiles so far and features two key players instead of one. Perhaps this dual focus comes just in time for those of you who insist that the real thing holding you back is *other people*.

The Issue: Failure of Vision

The Company: A New York Brokerage House, Compliance Division
The Players: David R., 37; Sylvia A., 44

In the wake of 9/11, stockbrokers have faced new regulations and greater scrutiny to prevent terrorists from surreptitiously using them to launder money. This particular firm had been relying on old technology and insufficiently skilled labor to report suspicious activity to the government. Recently, after a government audit, they'd received a failing grade for their reports and were given a short time to turn the situation around.

The stakes were enormous. No other firm even near their size had yet been penalized, but a much smaller institution had just been fined $40 million. Beyond the prospect of an unprecedented fine, the company also faced the possibility of a long-term ban from key types of trading, which could end up costing billions (not to mention the potential homeland-security risks if the job wasn't done right). To top it off, government representatives were only allowed to tell the company what they were doing wrong, not how to fix the problem. The solution had to come from within.

At first glance, based on what I've presented so far, the solution might seem obvious: purchase better technology and provide adequate staff training. What I've left out, however, is the emotional component of the story, and this is where our two high-ranking managers come in.

Sylvia was in charge of the entire compliance division for the firm, which included far more than this particular type of reporting. Throughout twenty years of consistent promotion at the company, she'd garnered a reputation for ruthless but profitable cost cutting. A salary in the high six figures to go along with her cardiologist husband's income meant that Sylvia was pretty much set for life. The only missing piece for her was peace of mind, which she'd been chasing since early childhood. One of three sisters, Sylvia revered her father, an Oklahoma oilman who'd always wanted a boy. He taught his girls never to be weak and, even more importantly, never to be seen so. In truth, however, he believed that women were made weak, and Sylvia had spent most of her life trying to prove him wrong.

Sylvia wasn't my client. I learned some of her bio while consulting with the company, and the rest of it after my work there was done. While introspection wasn't Sylvia's forte, she was forced into it during company-mandated coaching to soften what her colleagues considered an unacceptably gruff management style. The coaching had made a big difference, yet she still had a ways to go. In tackling the reporting fiasco, her main method was to poach David, a renowned problem solver, from another division of the firm. She granted David a hefty salary and basically said, "Fix this."

David was my client. He had an effervescent manner that reminded me of "Zorba the Greek," and that often needed to be dampened down in a corporate context. I'd worked with David before as an executive coaching client on the West Coast. To take the job Sylvia offered, he uprooted his wife and two middle-school daughters from San Diego and resettled with them in the New Jersey suburbs. They weren't happy about it, but the opportunity won out. David's first task as head of the reporting department was to identify and purchase state-of-the-art financial-tracking technology. His second task was to assess the retrainability of the current staff. It was here that he encountered serious institutional resistance.

Across the board, his staff of seventy-five functioned in a pre-9/11 mind-set, handling their reports like widgets instead of paying them the close scrutiny that terrorism prevention demanded. Previously they'd been taught to follow orders and ask no questions. Now, encouraged to become nimble, creative entrepreneurs, they balked. When pushed, they fell back on an attitude of "None of this is our fault. Let's just keep doing what we've always done."

David worked with the human resources department of the company to develop fresh job-specific curricula. Still, months after implementing it, the old-school culture of the division remained stubbornly intact. That's when David contacted me again, interested in putting together some powerful "offsites," daylong training events that would finally get across the urgent need for change.

I began the project by distributing confidential questionnaires to the staff about their overall job satisfaction and enthusiasm. The questionnaire results, along with the first offsite, led me to a dire assessment. Most of the staff lacked the education, experience, and inclination to perform their newly empowered "first line of defense" function. For the majority, the job was nothing more than a paycheck.

David agreed with my assessment. He presented Sylvia with two options: (1) retrain as much of the staff as possible in a longer, more rigorous way, recognizing that many still wouldn't be able to cut it; or (2) reassign or let go the whole team and bring in new people who were truly motivated and qualified.

Sylvia chose neither option, considering them both way too expensive. She urged David to continue with the same staff and with less extensive retraining, hopeful that the department's new software, just now fully implemented, would do the trick. David knew this wasn't the case, since proper use of the software depended on a high level of user sophistication, but for the time being he decided to keep quiet. It was too soon to make a scene, he thought, and he'd be in a much better position to push the issue when the software provided no salvation.

Three months later, when the software's limitations were abundantly clear, David decided the time was right. But the showdown between him and Sylvia wasn't pretty. David's position was firm—you brought me here to do a job, and I need significantly more resources to succeed. Sylvia's position was equally firm—there's a cheaper way. There has to be. If you haven't found it yet, that's your failure. Following this pronouncement, voices rose. So did heartbeats. In the end neither Sylvia nor David grew overtly hostile, but they both came close.

After this showdown David asked me for some counseling outside the office. He saw himself in a real bind, longing to beg for his old job back, pack up the family, and return to San Diego posthaste. But that was out of the question, he told me, because his kids were finally settled in to their new school and would revolt if they had to move all over again. Plus, many in senior management at the firm would see him as a quitter, and he wasn't willing to let that happen.

David also mused about blowing the whistle to the government auditors, letting them know the full story and therefore escaping blame. This would portray Sylvia for what he thought she truly was, an egomaniacal hatchet woman who cared nothing about the company or the country, just her own reputation. But whistle-blowing was out of the question, too, because after fourteen years David was loyal to his employer. Additionally, he knew that such a move would amount to career suicide. And if he did just walk away, that would lead to the loss of everything he'd worked so hard for, a huge hit in self-esteem, and sudden financial peril.

Due to our previous work together, David already understood the tools of this book and had lots of experience putting them to use. So I reminded him that if contracted, we can't trust ourselves to see things clearly and make good decisions. Was this happening to him? I suggested that we put our tools to work and find out.

So far he'd identified two possible but untenable courses of action. Now I asked him to imagine pursuing each, one after the other, in a way similar to Randall's exploration of his adrenaline rush (see page 118). First we looked at quitting and returning to San Diego. David saw the worst-case scenario with this option would be his daughters' growing to hate him. And how would that make him feel? David zeroed in on "all-encompassing guilt," a storm that I then asked him to weather. Guilt, for him, was a wrenching tug through his rib cage, as if he were literally being turned inside out. When this passed after a couple of minutes, a mild state of expansion ensued. David realized that, while excruciating, he could indeed endure such a scenario in real life. It would be possible to explain to his girls the complex set of needs and values that had led to this choice, and hopefully in time they would come to understand and forgive him.

Next we looked at whistle-blowing. David identified two worst-case scenarios here, being labeled a traitor by his peers and ultimately going broke. We took these scenarios one at a time. Being labeled a traitor created a feeling of self-loathing. This took awhile to clarify, because there were also a lot of inner voices in David that rose up to justify whistle-blowing and therefore claim that his self-loathing wasn't valid or acceptable. Soon enough, however, David was able just to let the self-loathing swirl through his chest and stomach, which in turn allowed it to yield to expansion and the recognition that, if necessary, he could indeed tolerate this outcome.

Regarding possible financial ruin, David saw the emotional cost as feeling like a "total loser." When he conjured this emotion, it brought up an image of him cold and homeless on a dirty street, curled up in a ball as all the "important people" walked by in disgust. Physically, the emotion centered at the back of his throat like a searing liquid. In a minute or two, both the image and the sensation dissolved. In their place arose a kind of quiet sadness, not altogether desirable yet still soft and open. From here David understood that "total loser" wouldn't be objectively true, permanent, or incapacitating, but instead just a tolerable and transient state.

Okay, so where were we now? David said that weathering these multiple storms allowed him to sense viscerally that he would end up okay if forced to make either of these objectionable choices. But then something entirely different happened. Freed of his resistance-induced blind spot, David began to see another option. Even though he reported directly to Sylvia, and even though his company frowned on end runs, in an extreme case like this David could appeal all the way to the CEO's office. Just this sudden recognition that another choice was possible caused David to heave a giant sigh of relief.

But we didn't stop there. I invited David to revisit his judgment of Sylvia conceived out of upset and to view her with clearer, more expansive eyes. At first he protested, telling me that he'd already been down this road. He'd studied the times of day when she was most receptive to new ideas or bad news. He'd discerned the tones of voice that set her at ease, as well as the ones that raised her ire. He'd even got his hands, somehow, on part of the evaluation from her compulsory coaching sessions. With all this, David considered himself a near expert on Sylvia's MO.

Deferring to this research, I asked David what the worst-case scenario was for Sylvia in regard to their mutual predicament. He thought about it and then said, "Losing her reputation." And how would that make her feel, I wondered. "Well," David said, "I guess I don't really know."

Before David appealed to the CEO, I suggested that he take Sylvia to lunch and find out. Just as David's emotional resistance had created his inability to see the complete picture, perhaps Sylvia was in the same boat. Perhaps understanding the emotional storm that *she* was desperate to avoid would point toward an additional course of action.

David took me up on this suggestion and used nearly all his people skills to deflect Sylvia's initial suspicion about the purpose of their meeting. During the lunch, he shared openly about the emotional difficulties that his whole family had faced during their speedy transcontinental move. Sylvia sympathized and seemed relieved not to be talking about their conflict. Encouraged but without knowing about the gold that he was about to strike, David described how being the son of an absentee father made him especially concerned with fostering healthy daughters who felt really good about themselves. Hearing this, Sylvia offered just enough about her own family background for David to glean that the feeling of weakness was her emotional Achilles heel. They each left the lunch feeling a little less distrustful, and David suddenly had a new plan.

It was clear to him now that Sylvia hadn't been unwilling, but instead unable, to see key pieces of the reporting puzzle. Beyond just preserving her reputation, she had an emotional need to handle the current crisis, as well any other, in a way that made her feel powerful and competent— anything but weak. Even though David didn't share this concern, he was easily able to find emotional correlates for it inside himself. Empathizing in this way led him not only to understand Sylvia's resistance more fully but also to adjust for it deftly.

David wrote a new, comprehensive memo that to an untrained eye would have looked similar to his last one. But this memo was designed to address Sylvia's blind spots directly. In a nonconfrontational manner he added exhaustive detail to buttress points that other readers would have accepted without question. Rather than focus solely on keeping costs to a minimum, which a more superficial reading of Sylvia would have dictated and which she herself would have consciously preferred, David argued that spending liberally in the short term would save significantly over the long haul.

More important, he highlighted that it would take great vision, and especially *strength*, to sell this approach companywide. Furthermore, bucking the likely resistance from penny-pinching investors and shareholders would lead the firm to a new reputation for bold innovation and raise the bar for the whole industry. Finally, failing to take this approach would not only lead to staggering financial losses, for which the compliance division would be directly responsible, but would also create a PR nightmare in which the firm would become a poster child for greed, cruelty, and cowardice—in other words, the next Enron.

Taking advantage of his newly gained camaraderie with Sylvia, David walked her through the report in person, section by section. He took great care to gauge not only her verbal cues but also her body language. A couple of times, when he thought she was hardening, David slowed down, lowered his voice, and sat down right beside her. Soon they saw eye to eye. Sylvia agreed with the very same proposals she'd vetoed previously. In addition, remarkably, she helped David devise a strategy to sell the solution in-house.

Best of all, it worked. No quitting, whistle-blowing, or end runs were required. Within eighteen months the company was back in the government's good graces and received significant PR points for tackling the problem head-on and becoming an exemplary partner in terrorism prevention.

Key Refinements

THE FORK IN THE ROAD

Whenever you're at a difficult crossroads, whether at work or elsewhere, a vital question to ask is: am I about to choose from resistance or acceptance? Choosing from resistance means that you're going in one direction to avoid the emotional consequences of going in the other. This isn't bad or wrong, but it does mean, based on the nature of resistance, that you'll be visiting that temporarily avoided emotion farther along the road. Choosing from acceptance means that you've "felt into" the worst-case scenarios for all possible directions, have expanded into an acceptance of the emotions they'll likely elicit, and are therefore reasonably confident that your decision-making process isn't motivated by emotional defense.

If it seems likely that your decision-making process contains some resistance, and you're willing to investigate further, do what David did. Imagine your way through a worst-case scenario for all the identified options. In this case, rather than discovering emotional resistance that's already been keeping you stuck, what you're doing

FORK IN THE ROAD

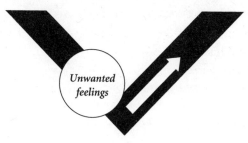

Choosing from resistance

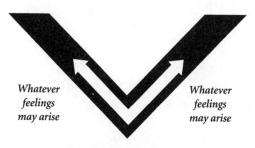

Choosing from acceptance

FIGURE 9

is ensuring *in advance* that this won't occur. If the process is either rough or halting, simply apply any or all of the specialized techniques and refinements we've covered previously. They work just as well in this precautionary way as they do when damage has already been done.

It's important to note what happened to David when he employed emotional connection at the fork in his own personal road. Rather than gaining clarity about which path to choose, as often occurs, David's expansion led him to notice a different path altogether. This is common too. When we free ourselves from resistant thinking and bring the three main aspects of our mind into harmony, blind spots lift, and inspiration appears. On page 111 we looked briefly at the importance of moving from a framework of either/or to both/and. At a fork in the road, emotional connection takes us one step further, allowing us to move from either/or to many/more.

CORE CONCEPT

When emotional connection brings our mind into harmony, new ideas and choices naturally arise.

TACTICAL EMPATHY

In the introduction, I mentioned that emotional intelligence entered the public conversation during the nineties with Daniel Goleman's book of the same name. Goleman's newest book is called *Social Intelligence,* and in it he argues that our facility with emotions isn't complete until we can feel not just our own but also others'. He identifies empathy as an essential life skill for each of us personally and for the planet's very survival as well. Fortunately, our aptitudes for emotional connection and empathy develop roughly in tandem. The more we can feel our own feelings directly, without resistance or filters, the better able we can discern those same feelings in virtually everyone we encounter.

The benefits of empathy are many, but from David's example we can glean one in particular. Empathizing with coworkers helps us immeasurably in reaching our goals and also in doing so more quickly and efficiently. David almost certainly would not have been able to win Sylvia as an ally without feeling how the whole issue was living inside her. Once he was willing, it took just a slight shift in emphasis to yield major results.

In some cases we can empathize straightaway, either because the other people involved reveal their emotions to us or because we intuitively get it. On the whole, however, it's not advisable to assume how anyone else is feeling. The best approach is to ask first, listen carefully, and only then attempt to empathize.

When you do ask, often the question will be deflected. People rarely share their vulnerable feelings without a real sense of affinity and safety. Because the ultracompetitive world of business doesn't usually foster such affinity and safety, it takes great care to engage with coworkers in this way. David, as I mentioned, needed all his own people skills to draw Sylvia into the emotional realm. Even then, he still required a little luck to gain his key empathetic insight.

The communication methods necessary to maximize empathy are outside the scope of this discussion (see page 150 for a little more on the subject), but the important thing to underline is the element of choice involved. While sometimes empathy comes unbidden, most of the time it's the result of our decision to resonate with someone else's emotional experience. Whenever we make that decision, what allows us to implement it successfully is connecting to the parallel emotional experience within ourselves. In other words, we can't literally feel another person's emotions, but it's by feeling those same emotions internally that we establish empathetic resonance.

Such resonance is what distinguishes tactical empathy from manipulation. When we're connected to our own feelings and to the feelings of those around us, we make decisions that are for the most part wise and humane.

CORE CONCEPT

Emotional connection, internally and with others, leads to wise, humane decisions.

Emotional disconnection, on the other hand, usually leads to decisions that are more about personal gain than the greater good.*
This would have been the case for David if he'd understood only

---

*The major exception to this principle, of course, are high-pressure jobs such as paramedic or police officer that require our emotional responses to be set aside while in the line of duty.

Sylvia's emotional constitution from the outside rather than taking the extra step of connecting to it within. Such manipulation, in my experience, leads to bad blood and eventually backfires. Yet more important, for the majority of us who strive to do well *and* good, manipulative disconnection robs us of our moral compass. To discern our deepest convictions, and to act upon them, we must be emotionally and empathetically adept.

THE EMOTIONAL AUDIT

While reading the story of David and Sylvia, it's possible to doubt that emotions, resistance, and personal conflicts would play such a large role in key corporate decision making. It's easy to assume that a firm's management structure and oversight functions would mitigate the role of individuals and their issues. But anyone who ever actually worked in upper management will tell you otherwise. This is how it almost always happens. People pretend or even really believe that their points of view are solely strategic, motivated by the bottom line, while their true motivations are actually to a great degree emotional.

Conversely, no one denies the existence or centrality of organizational politics. It's a given that people struggle for power and control in virtually every group situation. This is true whether that struggle is public, behind the scenes, or both. And here, too, emotions are key. People pursue power and control primarily to cultivate the feelings of satisfaction they believe will ensue. Their emotional drives and resistances, usually unconscious, are what dictate their political maneuverings.

Therefore, in every workplace emotions are at the heart of how individual and collective goals are both formulated and applied. Real, lasting success dictates that we not only acknowledge this but also foster emotional connection and empathy as vital professional skills. This is just as true at a school, church, or charity as it is at a multinational corporation. Beyond giving emotions their due and learning to engage with them proficiently, we must also address the emotional *culture* of any collective endeavor.

Every group has a feel to it. That feel may be sober, exciting, driven, formal, casual, aggressive, or cautious. The list is endless and includes all sorts of combinations. Take a moment and think about each group in which you're involved. What does it feel like? What feeling does it promote? Does it succeed in creating such an emotional culture? Does it pay lip service to one kind of feeling while actually creating another? What emotions *aren't* welcome in the group? When and how does this emotional resistance affect and hamper the group's mission?

The above questions constitute an emotional audit. An emotional audit can be done on one's own, among two partners, within a small department, a big division, and even a whole company. Both up and down the chain of command, the emotional culture at one level of a group can produce ripple effects for all the others. It's difficult to overemphasize the importance and advantage of assessing an organization in this way. Personally, whenever hired as a consultant, I make sure that some form of an emotional audit is the first service my team provides.

In working with David and his department, I first administered an emotional audit in the form of a questionnaire, just one of many tools available to get the job done. Later, David and I also performed an unofficial audit of his firm's overall emotional culture in determining whether an end run to top executives was the best strategy. It turned out that feelings of unity and trust were highly promoted company-wide. To a large extent this was just internal propaganda rather than standard operating procedure, but it still had the potential to diminish David's prospects for a full, impartial hearing if he appeared at all disloyal to his superior. This recognition, in part, was behind my suggestion that David keep looking for additional options.

Here's a good way to sum up this key refinement: everything we've covered so far in relation to individuals pertains equally to groups. Emotional resistance is the one thing holding groups back from achieving their greatest possible results. An emotional audit is an essential first step in bringing those results about.

PRACTICAL TIP

An emotional audit is an essential first step for any group seeking to reach its peak potential.

It enables a group or individuals within that group to identify their best next steps with confidence and then implement them with the least likely interference.

The Issue: Inability to Change Careers
Fran R.—*System Administrator, 31, Tuscaloosa, Alabama*

After the long and intricate profile of David and Sylvia, let's take a look at some briefer, more straightforward examples of emotional connection. First there's Fran, who worked her way up to a stable position, good salary, and generous benefits at a global telecom company. The only problem was that Fran fell into her sys-admin position straight out of college, and it wasn't what she really wanted to do. Ever since she saw Holly Hunter in the film *Broadcast News*, Fran dreamed of becoming a TV producer.

Originally, friends and family scared Fran off with talk of how cutthroat the media business can be, but the dream never died, and she realized that her window for starting over at the bottom was soon about to close. Every time she imagined throwing away the relative security of her current career track, however, Fran would freeze. This, of course, was her flinch.

Fran and I worked together for only one session. During that session, she saw that her worst-case scenario was never graduating out of the mailroom at some small local affiliate. Such an outcome, she realized, would make her feel stupid, first for having given up so many blessings in leaving her old career, and then again for not having what it takes to succeed in her new one.

As Fran began to weather that storm of feeling stupid, her face, neck, and shoulders flushed. Then the emotion shifted to anger, in her belly, at having been brainwashed into such timidity for so many years.

Soon the anger shifted as well, leaving Fran with a feeling of failure, which weighed heavily from her chest downward. Next, the failure morphed into loss, and that brought a few tears. Fran wiped the tears away, blew her nose, and then settled back into a philosophical pose. "Now," she told me, "I just feel resigned. Like . . . oh well, at least I tried. It's not so bad, really. I mean it's way better than never having given it a shot."

A few months later, after repeating as necessary a few times, Fran was finally able to muster up her courage and quit. She used her savings to bankroll a six-month, unpaid internship at a Tuscaloosa TV station. After that, Fran took a minimum-wage job there as a production assistant, during which she felt "jazzed" just to be pulling cable and adjusting the teleprompter. Today she's an associate producer at the same station, making one-third the salary of her previous job. Yet she remains satisfied, thrilled even, to have made the career transition before it was too late. Even if she never graduates to the national level, Fran insists, the decision to pursue her dream job will still remain worthwhile.

Key Refinement

MUTABILITY

Emotions change. When you weather any storm or simply apply the 2 X 2 process to become emotionally present during ordinary times, you find almost immediately that feelings can seamlessly transform into one another. Mourning can become peace, envy can become appreciation, and any other emotion can either gradually or suddenly be replaced within your bodily awareness by another one waiting in line.

While we've seen numerous examples previously of physical sensations changing and of emotions flowing throughout different parts of the body on their way to final release, Fran's story is the first time that an important breakthrough required staying present throughout a veritable emotional parade. Such a parade will likely be common as you deepen your own emotional awareness. Yet a shifting array of emotions requires nothing truly different than the skills we've already covered. Just 2 X 2 those feelings into an expanded state, and keep noticing for a little longer than usual. This extra time will ensure that any lingering feelings have a chance to bring up the rear and gain the benefit of your equal and complete attention.

Fran's story also highlights something we all already know well—it's possible to have many different emotions, and even conflicting ones, about the same issue. This only becomes a problem if we decide it is, and if we therefore slip into a judging or either/or state. When this happens, we may weather only part of the storm while leaving another important part blustering inside. Luckily for Fran, she didn't have any resistance to feeling stupidity, anger, failure, loss, and resignation, one right after the other in quick succession. This is precisely what made her a "one appointment wonder," needing no additional outside assistance in finally breaking through her block.

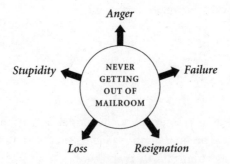

**Fran's worst-case scenario, like many situations,
elicits multiple and even conflicting emotions.**

FIGURE 10

Just as a reminder, working with multiple emotions doesn't require you to name each and every one. Sometimes they move so fast that it's not even possible to identify them individually. Attempting to do so at such moments is counterproductive and can dam up an otherwise robust flow.

While we're on the subject of emotional mutability, it's a good time to address a common obstacle to complete connection. When attempting to 2 X 2, many people proclaim, "I'm not just feeling one emotion. A bunch of them are happening all at once." This, however, rarely occurs. It only seems that way from a distance and with a quick glance—like looking at an anthill while passing by and noting only a homogenous blob. As noted before, slowing down and getting microscopic with any anthill will begin to reveal its activities in careful coordination and sequence. So if you seem to be feeling more than one thing at a time, just slow down further and pay a little more attention. You'll usually find that there are indeed multiple emotions present, but that they're following one another almost imperceptibly.

This point about emotions only arising single file was driven home to me during my years in the entertainment industry. When directing the actor Jason Alexander in a scene of my film, *Sexual Healing,* I told him to deliver a speech with a mixture of anger and sadness. Reluctantly, he agreed, and as I watched his facial expressions, I couldn't make out anything at all. Then Jason took me aside gently and suggested that he deliver the first lines of the speech with anger, then quickly shift to sadness midway through. It worked like a charm, and the sequence of expressions on his face was both moving and richly distinct.

The Issue: Project Paralysis
Hans B.—Research Physicist, 51, Los Alamos, New Mexico

Hans had two decades under his belt at one of the world's leading scientific laboratories. Accomplished and respected, he was experiencing a stubborn block in meeting an important grant-proposal deadline. Even though he had already gathered the necessary data and put it all together in outline form, the actual writing just wasn't happening. Hans was confused and frustrated, especially since he usually cranked out such proposals on virtual automatic pilot.

In working with Hans, I tried all the tools in the toolbox. None made much of a dent, and the deadline was fast approaching. Even finding the flinch and cutting to the chase came up short, because although Hans wanted this particular grant, he would also have been perfectly fine without it. Therefore, there was no real storm for him to weather.

I decided to set the toolbox aside for a moment and simply talk with Hans. I learned that in preliminary reviews with the granting agency, an administrator had suggested that Hans alter his research methods in a small and relatively insignificant way. When Hans told me this, he unconsciously hunched his shoulders and brought one leg up on his chair. It seemed to bother him more than his casual tone was letting on. Taking this as a clue, I asked Hans what it felt like to have his study interfered with. At first he tried to brush off the whole thing but then admitted that it griped him.

Next, I suggested that Hans use the posture-movement-sound techniques (pages 45–47) to exaggerate that feeling of being griped. When he did, this led him to scowl, shake his fists, and snarl like an animal ready to pounce. I encouraged Hans to stay with this exaggerated emotion and inquired whether he remembered ever feeling like it in the past. After a few moments he reported that it came up a lot during playtime squabbles with his older brother. This brother was bossy, a bully, and often drained their games of fun. When I probed a little further, Hans told me that his usual response was to quit in a huff and stomp away, retreating into a book or some other solitary activity.

Did this seem at all relevant to his current situation, I asked. Hans drew an immediate parallel. "I won't write the proposal because that guy changed the rules on me. I don't like the game anymore. I'm taking all my marbles and going home." It sounded right to me, but then Hans reconsidered. "That's stupid. You think this whole paralysis thing is related to some childhood tussles with my brother? From thirty years ago?" I reminded Hans that my own view mattered much less than what his emotions told him and that it's easy to lapse into judgment about such emotional responses when they seem inappropriate.

Hans understood, calmed down, and we agreed to see what would happen over the next few days. Sure enough, the grant proposal just poured right out. A couple of times he almost froze up, agitated by thoughts of his brother and the administrator, but a brief return to posture-movement-sound got the writing quickly back on track.

Key Refinements

EXAGGERATION

Every once in a while, even with lots of effort, the emotional dots just won't connect. It seems obvious in these cases that there's resistance afoot, but every attempt to break through comes up short. When this happens, it's often helpful to pretend that you're feeling much more intensely than you actually are. For Hans, this meant exaggerating the small annoyance with his grant administrator to the point of near absurdity. Only by flooding his system in this way was he able to bypass the paralysis that his conscious efforts at understanding had created. He could then shift, as the next refinement demonstrates, from our usual and more straightforward approaches to one that relies upon emotional association.

USING EXAGGERATION TO REVEAL AND FREE EMOTION

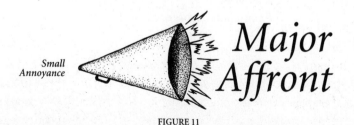

Small Annoyance

Major Affront

FIGURE 11

EMOTIONAL ASSOCIATION

Whenever we respond to a present-day situation in a mysterious, challenging way, the likely cause is that this event has stirred up the emotional dust of some previous, unresolved incident. Earlier, we discussed how it's unnecessary to go searching for those previous incidents and their corresponding emotions, because our very willingness to employ emotional connection in the here and now will naturally bring them to the surface. Sometimes, however, that process is stymied by our inability to initiate emotional connection regarding our *current* concern. That's what happened with Hans until his use of exaggeration opened things up a little and made it possible for him to associate his past and present annoyances. Once that happened, as you may have noticed, he didn't even need the 2 X 2 process to clear the old feelings. Much of the time this is the case with or without the use of exaggeration. The basic aha, along with the expansion it brings, is enough.

Most people move easily into the realm of emotional association by asking, *When have I felt this way before?* But if that question doesn't yield a helpful answer or you don't yet know what you're feeling, try asking, *What similar situations have I experienced before?* Identifying those situations and comparing them to what's happening right now can provide a shortcut to their common emotional content.

PRACTICAL TIP

**Emotional association can help you quickly
determine whether your current feelings are unduly
influenced by resistance from the past.**

Both versions of this question are standard features in many forms of therapy. The reason they require the participation of a therapist is because most clients haven't yet mastered the other practices presented here. Once you feel relatively proficient in those practices, however, you can almost always draw sufficient "juice" from emotional association on your own.

The Issue: A Personal Injustice

Kenneth T.—Bridge Builder, 41, Oakland, California

Kenneth was a man's man, well over six feet tall, broad shouldered and stern. He was lead construction engineer for a company building a new, earthquake-resistant bridge. At a crucial stage of the building process, Kenneth reported some structural-integrity issues to his boss, recommending a longer, costlier, but ultimately safer approach. His boss rejected Kenneth's recommendation, citing a looming deadline and assuring Kenneth that everything was up to snuff. Three months later their work failed a state transportation-department review. The company was forced to implement Kenneth's original suggestions after all, at a much higher cost than would have been incurred earlier.

Rather than accepting responsibility for his own misjudgment, the boss blamed Kenneth. He lied and passed the buck, insisting that Kenneth had never explained the situation accurately. Kenneth, for his part, hadn't bothered to document their earlier conversation and therefore wasn't able to defend himself. As a result he was demoted and forced to take a corresponding pay cut. Kenneth wanted to quit more than anything, but he couldn't afford losing health insurance because his eight-year-old daughter was seriously ill.

In our work together, Kenneth followed this story by describing the flare-up of an old back injury. At this point, he told me, it took prescription meds just to keep him on the job. We began by focusing on his pain, 2 X 2-ing it as with a contraction. It turned out that this pain *was* a contraction, at least in part, because after a few moments the pain gave way to an almost overwhelming rush of anger.

Kenneth's anger felt like a fire that spread outward from his chest. In his mind, he kept hearing the phrase, *"I'm going to kill that son of a bitch!"* This scared Kenneth and made him pause for a moment, uncertain it was healthy to give in to that kind of rage. I explained to him that feeling what's already present is actually the opposite of acting it out and that mental phrases can accompany emotions in the same harmless way that images do.

Convinced that it was safe to keep letting his anger flow, Kenneth dove back in. In a few moments, however, the anger shifted. Suddenly Kenneth seemed small and fragile and described an ache in his chest where the anger had just been. Using the 2 X 2 process caused the ache to intensify, and Kenneth closed his eyes as if to fight back tears. When he opened his eyes, they were indeed wet, and Kenneth looked away in embarrassment. After a few moments I asked him if he was familiar with this feeling. He wasn't. I guided him to stay connected with it for another long stretch.

"It's hurt," he realized. "Hurt to be wrongly accused . . . taken advantage of . . . and, I guess, not having any way to stand up for myself." Before continuing, I asked Kenneth what level of pain he was currently experiencing in his back. He checked, then paused to double-check. "None," he answered with surprise.

While Kenneth kept tracking his hurt, I discussed the way that some pain is actually somaticized emotion, meaning that the raw energy of unfelt feelings gets diverted into a bodily complaint. Frequently, such pain releases for good once its underlying emotion is accessed. A release of this kind may also just be temporary, but in these cases the 2 X 2 process can still act as a powerful pain reliever.

After another couple of minutes, Kenneth's hurt eased into what felt like a bigger, softer space beneath his ribs. I introduced Kenneth to the concept of protective and core emotion, noting that his anger was essentially a response to his hurt. Both had a place and a purpose, but the hurt was crucial. Any kind of anger management that didn't also address the hurt would be unsatisfying and incomplete. "Hurt management," in the form that Kenneth had just practiced, was actually the best way to make his situation tenable as long as he chose to stay with his current employer.

When I last checked in with Kenneth, he was indeed still at the same job. His daughter was recovering from a successful surgery and seemed to be out of the woods. Kenneth was beginning to look for other opportunities now that he could risk a gap in insurance coverage. In the meantime he gave himself a B- at hurt management, recognizing that it was the only thing allowing him to bear the daily encounters with his boss but also recognizing that it wasn't an easy fit with his macho persona. He found that 2 X 2 worked best for him in the steam room at his gym. There, safely obscured by all the mist, he could freely access his recurring hurt and let it gradually melt away.

Since he was in a self-evaluating mode, I asked Kenneth to assess the level of upset he currently experienced compared to when we'd first met in the previous month. He said that with the exception of a few bad days, it had gone from an 8 to a 4. Surprised at such positive results, and sharing Kenneth's own recognition that he'd never quite be the touchy-feely type, I asked him to consider bumping up his hurt management grade to A-. Sheepishly, he agreed.

Key Refinements

WORKING WITH PHYSICAL PAIN

In chapter 1, when first discussing the nature of emotion, I noted that there's no immediate way to determine the difference between a physical sensation and an emotion. I maintained that only sustained attention can produce a successful determination. What Kenneth's story tells us, in addition, is how interrelated sensation and emotion truly are. Connecting to any type of physical discomfort with the 2 X 2 process can quickly reveal the degree to which our discomfort has been *caused* by emotion. In these cases our resistance to the emotion in its original manifestation drives it into our subconscious. There, the emotion keeps up its campaign for our attention by resurfacing as a nasty ache. That's why 2 X 2, for at least five minutes, is a vital part of any truly holistic diagnosis for chronic or mysterious pain. There's never anything to lose from such bodily exploration, except often, as with Kenneth's back-injury flare-up, the pain itself.

Taking this approach a step further, I also recommend 2 X 2 for any pain that's obviously nonemotional, such as a simple cut or sprain. In these situations feeling the pain deeply and directly elucidates the way we feel *about* the pain, which in turn can liberate otherwise stuck emotions.

PRACTICAL TIP

Practicing 2 X 2 with physical pain is helpful whether or not emotions contributed to it in the first place.

Here's a personal example. The other night, while hastily chopping vegetables, I accidentally sliced my finger. The pain wasn't too bad, but I used the 2 X 2 process for a minute and was suddenly awash with frustration. My frustration was a response to the pressure I felt being long overdue on the manuscript of this very book! It seemed as if I didn't even have sufficient time to prepare and eat my meals and that so much rushing around in the kitchen had practically insured such an injury.

As I fully felt all that frustration and pressure, they soon began to diminish. It was clear to me, in a sudden flash, that there was no actual pressure at all. My editor was waiting patiently for the book, more than willing to allow me extra time in pursuit of a quality draft. Realizing this, I exhaled in such a long and gratifying way that it seemed as if I'd been holding my breath for days. Had I just cleaned and bandaged the cut, without any 2 X 2, I would have missed the opportunity to free myself of such self-created and debilitating tension.

PROTECTIVE VS. CORE EMOTIONS

With Fran's story about changing careers, we came to recognize that the flow of emotion toward expansion often includes not just one but many feelings. Kenneth's profile points out that the direction this multiple flow usually takes is from protective to core. A protective emotion, similar to a contraction, is meant to shield us from an initial, more threatening emotion that has already arisen. Knowing this, however, isn't enough to change it. Only when we actually allow the protective emotion to run its course can the core emotion then do the same.

No other emotion shows up more in this protective-core scenario than anger. As difficult as anger can be to experience, it has an empowering quality. It allows us to feel, if not in control of a situation, at least assertive about it. The entire range of vulnerable emotions, on the other hand—such as hurt, loss, abandonment, and grief—leaves us feeling defenseless and exposed.

PROTECTIVE EMOTIONS

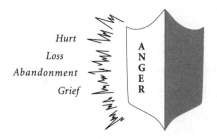

Hurt
Loss
Abandonment
Grief

A N G E R

Protective emotions shield us
from more threatening ones.

FIGURE 12

Exposure to core emotions is much more difficult than anger for most of us to tolerate. It can feel like we're being flayed alive or devoured whole. When a core emotion is indeed so vulnerable, our primitive minds won't even allow us to register it. In a split second after the painful event, we shift into fight mode. Anger becomes not just a shield but also a sword, whether we wield it against others or ourselves. The good news, however, is that no matter which of these ways our anger manifests, and no matter how overwhelming it seems at first, the 2 X 2 process quickly enables us to drop the sword and pursue more complete awareness.

This distinction between protective and core feelings doesn't change our working model of emotional connection or our understanding of how to apply it. But what it does provide is increased motivation to let vulnerable emotions have their full say. Feeling vulnerable emotions fully is what lets us expand fully and therefore experience all the subsequent benefits. These benefits are vital when a painful situation must be temporarily endured, like Kenneth's demotion, but also, and even more so, when we're ready to pursue proactive change.

The Issue: Downsizing

Tina A.—Vice President, Customer Support, 36,
Fairfax, Virginia

We began our workplace profiles with David, who was responsible for saving his company millions of dollars in potential losses and fines but had to overcome one resistant colleague to do so. We now end our workplace profiles with Tina, who was also required to save her company millions of dollars but had to confront *three hundred colleagues* to do so.

Over an eight-year period, Tina had built and nurtured an award-winning software call center. It's no exaggeration to say that she took a personal interest in all the people who staffed her center, as well as offering them flextime, telecommuting, and whatever else possible to promote their well-being and retention.

Then the ax fell for the call center, in the form of a well-regarded Mumbai, India, facility that offered to perform the same services at one-fourth the cost. At first Tina balked, searching long and hard for similar cost-cutting solutions to keep the call center Stateside. When none could be found, she signed the deal and seemed to be at peace, until racked in the days that followed by unexpected and debilitating guilt. Although the outsourcing was inevitable and clearly not Tina's fault, she still felt responsible for all the soon-to-be-jobless workers. These feelings would overwhelm her when she least expected it—during her son's soccer game, while out to dinner with her husband and friends, and even awakening her in the middle of the night from already-fitful sleep.

The worst part, from a professional standpoint, was that Tina suddenly couldn't focus. She hoped to make the best of a bad situation for her staff by attending to every last detail of the transition, but just the thought of all their faces upon hearing the news made it impossible for her even to *begin* such a plan.

Tina kept telling herself to keep a stiff upper lip, but that wasn't making a dent. Instead, she just grew angry and tense, taking it out on her family and only adding to the guilt. It was when she flirted with an old drinking habit that Tina became frightened enough to seek help.

When Tina shared this story with me, I was reminded of Gloria, the nearly burned-out lawyer who needed to stop repressing her emotions and find a healthy schedule for feeling them (page 24). I was also reminded of Kenneth, from the previous profile, who needed to get past his protective anger in order to befriend his more vulnerable core hurt. But beyond such comparisons, I sought the true nature of Tina's guilt, which seemed like an authentic and caring response, yet at the same time was incommensurate with the situation. After all, Tina's clarity that the downsizing wasn't her fault did nothing to stop the guilt from assailing her.

Since Tina's worst-case scenario had already materialized, along with its matching emotion, I asked her if she'd be willing to spend some time weathering the storm. She held back at first, protesting that weathering the storm was all she'd *been* doing, but I explained to her that vacillating back and forth between resistance and acceptance, and between protective emotions and their core undercurrents, wasn't the same as gentle, spacious 2 X 2. Sometimes all the feeling in the world won't create any significant expansion if it's not done in a patient and consistent manner. Furthermore, I encouraged Tina to pause the process at any time if it became too painful and then to decide whether to stop for good or to pinpoint and keep going. At that, Tina set aside her reservations and gave it a try.

Very quickly, Tina's guilt revealed itself in full, vulnerable splendor. As physical sensation, it was a pursing of the lips and a feeling of collapsing inward from her shoulders to hips. As image, it portrayed key scenes from her broken home growing up, with Tina desperately, precociously trying to bring about some peace. Tina also kept hearing phrases in her mind such as, "I have to make them happy again," and "This is all because of me." Within just a few minutes both Tina and I realized that the backlog of childhood guilt she carried was considerable and that while this first unadulterated version of 2 X 2 brought her a small amount of relief, she'd likely need to repeat the process a number of times over the next few weeks.

The problem, however, was that Tina didn't have a few weeks. In just days she was set to announce the outsourcing to her whole team. She needed, in her words, "not to be a wreck." We talked about staving off emotion temporarily with the "not now, later" approach, but I had the feeling Tina was a little too volatile for all that. It turned out I was right, and the morning after our session she threw a full-scale tantrum in her boss's office. She vented about the unfairness of it all, about government policies that discouraged companies from keeping jobs in the United States, and especially about the other divisions of the company that weren't forced to make anywhere near the same kind of drastic cuts.

Tina's boss, surprisingly, just listened. A grandfatherly type, he nodded compassionately, resonated with what she was going through, and helped her calm down to the point at which real discussion was possible. Then he asked her lots of open-ended questions about the situation and listened some more. Tina left this meeting feeling even guiltier, this time for raving so irresponsibly, especially to someone who didn't deserve it. That afternoon she went back and apologized. Her boss was having none of it. "I was just doing my job," he told her. (In our parlance this entailed a wonderful application of tactical empathy). Tina thanked him for his caring and also told him about our session the day before. He encouraged her to schedule another session with me before the upcoming announcement, and she did so right away.

In this session we did some more 2 X 2 but mostly talked about the idea of proportionate response. I explained that since our emotional-feedback system is influenced by both our personalities and our pasts, we often find ourselves experiencing feelings that seem overly intense for the situation at hand. Ideally, when this happens, we're able to create the time and space necessary to ride these emotions out. Although such emotions usually require a longer, rougher path to expansion, the 2 X 2 process still allows us to get there. But sometimes, as with Tina and her downsizing dilemma, there just isn't time to cultivate expansion, harmonize our brains, and benefit from the insight and wisdom that result. Sometimes, as well, we're just not wired, willing, or ready for "not now, later." As a result, what we're left with is a storm, a need to weather it as best as possible, and no assurance of clearing anytime soon.

Lingering storm and all, however, we can still act with vision and skill. The first step in doing so is to acknowledge that our emotional feedback for the current situation is skewed. Next, we recognize that this distortion is likely to remain for a stretch and do our best not to make it worse by resisting. Finally, we look past the feeling, even while having it, to form an appropriate and effective way forward.

Heading back to the office with all this in mind, Tina plunged into her work. The guilt still remained and assaulted her in racking bursts. She'd keep it at arm's length for as long as possible, then stop for a few minutes and briefly let it have her full attention. At one point Tina found herself crying, which wasn't acceptable given the office's open floor plan, so she fled to the bathroom and let her tears fall in the privacy of a stall.

Calibrating her guilt in this way was tricky and required a high degree of self-monitoring, but it also yielded immediate results. Tina brainstormed with surprising ease about ways to support her staff through the transition. Rather than merely resenting the other VPs, she now requested their involvement in finding division reassignments for as many call-center employees as possible. She fought for a tiered severance package that was fair at each level of seniority. Finally, she sat patiently outside the CEO's office till he could give her ten minutes, during which she wrangled a special retraining allowance for any laid-off employee who requested it.

By the time Tina made the official announcement to her team, word had already begun to leak out. There were some groans and tears, to be sure, but most people took it in stride. The meeting remained calm and civil, without a single employee trying to shoot the messenger. Instead, hearing about Tina's sincere regret and the elaborate steps that she'd taken to ease their transition, many of the team members broke into applause.

Key Refinement

PROPORTIONAL RESPONSE

There are rare times when it's inappropriate to feel. Such times call for conscious emotional repression. Most other times we need to feel, fully, in order to live our best lives. Between these two poles exist occurrences when we need to regulate our emotional connection, staying present to feelings yet also distancing from them in a mindful balance. That's what proportional response is all about.

Tina came to realize that her overwhelming guilt was neither accurate nor helpful feedback. Attempting to repress it tilted her toward unkind and self-destructive behavior. Attempting to feel it revealed a daunting Pandora's box within. Throughout these experiments, her mission stayed consistent—serve both her company and employees as well as possible. It turned out that the best way to provide such service was feeling the guilt enough to remain alert, focused, and creative but not enough to let it drag her down. Tina's response to the guilt was perfectly proportional. Though unavoidably difficult and unpleasant, it enabled her to reach peak performance during a complex, precarious time.

When the downsizing was all over, Tina continued to work through her reservoir of childhood guilt at a depth that created real healing but that would have been entirely inappropriate during the previous pressure cooker. In essence she developed her own refinement to "not now, later," which might be stated as "a little now, a lot later."

The elements of successful proportional response are as follows:

1. Make no decisions about how much to feel until you've actually allowed yourself to feel for a good few minutes. In other words, any assessment made from a place of emotional disconnection will be premature and unreliable.

2. If you have the time and space necessary, go ahead and feel everything that arises. In doing so, you'll be able to determine how much of your response is from the present and how much is from the past. You'll not only address any old wounds involved, but you'll also update your emotional-feedback system for more accurate results in the future.

3. If circumstances make it impossible to feel everything that arises, and if turning off the emotional spigot isn't a good option either, employ trial and error to identify the amount of emotional connection that lets you be your best.

4. Keep connecting to your emotions at that amount, and tend to the remainder as soon as possible.

Reading this, you may doubt that emotions can be regulated as with a thermostat. You may be much more used to shutting off completely or periodically turning things up full blast than you are with finding an emotional comfort zone. Indeed, proportional response is the most sophisticated emotional technique I've presented.

PRACTICAL TIP

**Experiment with proportional response only
after mastering the other applications of
2 X 2 throughout the book.**

It takes great awareness and skill, as well as plenty of practice to find a version that fits both you and the moment best. In fact, during particularly trying situations, you may find yourself alternating rapidly between complete emotional connection, "not now, later," *and* proportional response. With enough time and commitment, however, this all becomes second nature. Where once you found yourself thwarted by resistance, now you're graced with choice and freedom.

12

RELATIONSHIPS AND COMMUNICATION

So FAR OUR Profiles of Emotional Connection have looked at nine people who were victorious over challenges relating to addiction, compulsion, and the workplace. No matter how private these victories were, they inevitably affected not just the individuals achieving them but also those around them. One profile, that of David and his struggles with Sylvia, made this collective benefit of emotional connection explicit. But David and Sylvia only scratched the surface of this benefit because emotions almost never exist in a personal vacuum. Most feelings arise to provide internal feedback about our external environment, and as long as that environment includes other people, our emotional lives will forever be social.

In any social context no one is immune from the impact of another's emotional resistance. When that resistance is overcome, everyone benefits. Often, how each individual in a group deals with emotions is contagious. This ripple effect can quickly lift the whole group up or just as quickly bring it down.

To best demonstrate that ripple effect in this chapter, we'll examine a small social network with a family at its center. Rather than focusing on one member at a time, we'll track the impact of emotional connection and disconnection across the whole network, interlacing our key refinements along the way. For an easy-reference summary of the players, their roles, and their impact on one another, consult the diagrams on pages 161 and 163.

Lisa, a forty-two-year-old resident of suburban Denver, was my client in this story and the source for most of the details to follow. Tall, outdoorsy, Lisa had bright red hair and an easy smile. Just after Lisa was born, her father divorced her mother and then pretty much disappeared while tending to a second family. This left Lisa with a great abandonment wound regarding men, particularly because her father seemed to choose his other kids over her. But what happened between Lisa and her mother was even more damaging. Lisa's mother was needy, demanding, and immature, more of a perpetual child than an adult. Her resistance to feeling abandoned, lonely, and helpless caused her to lean inappropriately on her daughter for all kinds of support, depriving Lisa of the space and separation any child needs to create a distinct and whole identity.

As a result of this upbringing, Lisa possessed an unusual combination of relationship traits. With all of her romantic partners she was clingy, desperate not to be left. But she also needed lots of alone time and would shut down whenever pressured for greater contact. In fact, she couldn't clearly distinguish a legitimate desire for togetherness and truly overbearing behavior. No matter how skillfully presented, and no matter which partner it came from, Lisa experienced every request for greater intimacy as an intolerable demand.

Lisa's resistance to feelings of abandonment and inundation were the one thing holding her back from creating a healthy, lasting relationship. Her resistance was also a perfect magnet for Bob, forty-three, the lanky, soft-spoken man she eventually married. Bob's parents stayed together, but they were both alcoholics. His father, a poor and frustrated actor, drank mostly to avoid feeling useless. His mother, devastated not to be living the "good life" she'd counted on, drank mostly to avoid feeling deprived. Their household was loud, combative, and volatile. This left Bob with a powerful craving for stability and peace. The one thing holding him back from a healthy, lasting relationship was his resistance to emotional turmoil.

On the surface, what drew Lisa and Bob together was their great chemistry. They liked many of the same things, shared a sarcastic sense of humor, and were compatible sexually. Underneath the surface, what drew Lisa and Bob together was the way they would push each other's buttons so perfectly. In one version, Lisa's clinginess would make Bob distant. The more dramatically she clung, the more distant and disapproving he'd become, creating a worst-case scenario for them both. In another version, Lisa's long stints in her shell would feel disruptive and unstable to Bob. He'd try to woo her back, which would only send her deeper into isolation.

Here was Lisa's main complaint: When I want more from Bob, he gives me less. When I need space from Bob, he smothers me.

Here was Bob's main complaint: Lisa wants us to be either joined at the hip or be like strangers. As soon as we find some middle ground, she always makes a scene.

Such complaints may seem relatively minor and easily addressed. Yet as we've covered previously, resistance creates huge blind spots. Even if solutions make logical sense, they won't work under fire unless there's enough corresponding expansion to support them. Lisa and Bob tried unsuccessfully to make progress both with couples therapy and pastoral counseling. They were unsatisfied, unhappy, and stuck.

Key Refinement

BUTTON POWER

It's natural not to like having our buttons pushed. It's natural to avoid the people who do it or to steel ourselves for battle with those we can't avoid. Yet when seeking emotional connection, both internally and with those who surround us, every button pushing is a gift. When at our best, we even *look forward* to the next time it happens. Why? Because nothing else can highlight our resistance as efficiently and therefore lead to the feelings that free us.

As the most insightful relationship theories make clear, we unconsciously seek out those who torment us for the illumination only they can provide. These people are the teeth to match our wounds, recalling Tynan's words, but this time with a positive spin. Lisa and Bob thought they were a great couple, at first, because of how well they got along. But the real reason they were a great couple was because of how completely they drove each other crazy.

PRACTICAL TIP

The best romantic partners understand that the ways they drive each other crazy provide a unique road map to personal and relationship freedom.

When your buttons are pushed and you remember to apply the 2 X 2 process, either right at that moment or as soon as possible thereafter, the results are likely to be quick and pronounced. Sometimes, years of resistance unclench in just a few moments. Backlogged emotions come surging through. Powerful insights appear. Expansive well-being takes hold in what were previously intolerable situations. Of course you still may have to repeat as necessary, and that may even mean daily, but now there's a lightness to the whole enterprise. You might find yourself thinking, *Oh, there's that button again. It's almost funny how predictable it is.*

When I met them, Lisa and Bob weren't yet able to take advantage of the opportunities that their mutual button pushing provided. But they weren't willing to give up on their marriage either. That was primarily because of their sixteen-year-old daughter, Abby, who was tall and thin like both of her parents and sported Lisa's bright red hair. Ever since they could remember, Abby was a brilliant yet difficult child. Fiercely independent and rebellious, Abby fought for her way with extreme displays of emotion. From moment to moment she could shift from irate to needy to downright unreachable. Her personality, with its blend of chaos and withdrawal, was seemingly designed to push both her parents' buttons with equal and brutal efficiency.

Lisa wanted desperately to save Abby from the same penchant for isolation she was painfully aware of in herself. But she couldn't keep from responding to it with a parental style that was intrusive, nagging, and a lot like what she'd once endured. Bob recoiled viscerally at Abby's fits, especially when they accompanied his wife's dramas, and this came across as unspoken but fuming disapproval. He was like a volcano, always about to blow but holding himself in check to avoid a reprise of his own explosive upbringing.

All this was difficult enough for the trio during Abby's childhood, but when she hit adolescence, things spiraled out of control. The more Abby disregarded all the rules her parents put forth, as well as the punishments that followed her transgressions, the more guilty and inadequate Lisa and Bob felt. Out of resistance to these feelings, Lisa and Bob clamped down harder, which only served to make things worse. They knew that the next few years were crucial in Abby's development and provided the last real chance they would have to make a positive impact. Yet here, just as in their own relationship, they both felt utterly stuck.

From Abby's perspective, her parents were always trying to tell her what to do while their own lives were a mess. She saw her mother as "always in my face." She saw her father as "mean, weak, afraid to stand up and make some noise." Underneath Abby's teenage bravado, however, it was also easy to sense strong need. From her mother, she craved autonomy and respect. From her father, she longed for safety and acceptance in a form that wouldn't be so shaken by all her tantrums and moods.

Abby's resistance to inundation and disapproval was holding her back from discovering an authentic identity rather than one shaped in reactive opposition to her parents. Her fiery displays were all born of this resistance rather than from the core emotions hidden beneath. As yet, she wasn't aware what those emotions were or even that they existed. All she knew for sure was that it felt really good, like an antidote to her home life, to be praised and adored. And that's what sent Abby head-long into the arms of Ike, a troubled eighteen-year-old dropout who was by no means her intellectual equal but was convinced she could do no wrong.

At this point in the development of our social network, we've looked at three generations of a family—Lisa and Bob, as well as their parents and daughter. We've seen how emotional resistance plays a role both within and between generations. We've also glimpsed the way that emotional lives don't just intersect, but overlap. It would be impossible to understand the individual emotional makeup of Lisa, Bob, or Abby without paying attention to their overall family legacy. Simultaneously, all three of them were resisting, infecting, experiencing, and expressing emotional aspects of one another.

CORE CONCEPT

In any social network, the members all resist, infect, experience, and express emotional aspects of one another.

Soon, we'll find out what happens to this family when emotional connection takes hold. But first, let's add one more member to our network.

Lisa and Bob first met at chiropractic school. Once they'd graduated and gained separate professional experience in a variety of offices, it was time for them to join forces. Without much money to invest, they chose to become junior partners in the practice of Quentin. Ruddy and warm, fifty-nine-year-old Quentin had recently been widowed and was looking forward to retirement. The plan was for a gradual transition over a number of years, during which Lisa and Bob would grow the practice and assume primary responsibility for it. Then, at a mutually agreed-upon time, Lisa and Bob would buy out Quentin's third of the practice, and the office would be theirs.

In the beginning the plan worked perfectly. Quentin had a lot of wisdom to share about the everyday operation of this type of business, while Lisa and Bob provided a big jolt of youthful enthusiasm. What made the partnership thrive even more was Quentin's great love for Abby. They bonded when she was very young, and he bestowed her with gifts and affection as if she were his own granddaughter.

Midway through the partnership, Quentin took a fall on the ski slopes that required two surgeries. His bones healed imperfectly and left him with terrible, chronic pain. In a short spell he went from cheerful to morose and could only come to work with the aid of OxyContin. Soon he was addicted, and this added a level of secrecy and unreliability to his deteriorating demeanor. Plus, since his health insurance didn't cover many of the bills, he had to deplete his retirement accounts to pay them. As a result, Quentin would not be able to retire for the foreseeable future. This left him bitter and left Lisa and Bob without a clear

THE PLAYERS

LISA: *42, Bob's wife and Abby's mother*
Abandonment issues due to father's absence
Dependency issues due to mother's needs

BOB: *43, Lisa's husband and Abby's father*
Averse to conflict and emotional turmoil due to alcoholic parents

ABBY: *16, Lisa and Bob's daughter*
Independent, rebellious, emotionally dramatic
Longing for autonomy from Lisa and acceptance from Bob

IKE: *18, Abby's troubled and adoring boyfriend*

QUENTIN: *59, Lisa and Bob's business partner*
Special bond with Abby
Addiction to painkillers following ski accident

FIGURE 13

path to their own practice. Furthermore, Quentin's behavior was veering toward the unprofessional, causing patients to leave and revenues to plummet. Last but not least, many of Quentin's long-term patients were switching over to Lisa or Bob, which created more bad blood for the previously peaceful trio.

Can you guess, from what you already know about Lisa's and Bob's patterns of resistance, how they responded to this challenge? Lisa took the almost complete disappearance of the formerly loving version of Quentin as an abandonment. It was as if a second father had checked out on her. She did everything possible to make things better, to win back his affection, which included overlooking all kinds of inconsiderate and offensive behaviors. Predictably, however, Quentin appreciated none of Lisa's efforts and responded to her needy entreaties with even greater irritation. Bob, for his part, couldn't bear that his once-placid office had become an unpredictable war zone. He tried to keep a safe distance from Quentin and hide his disapproval but grew more visibly disgruntled with every passing day.

Bob blamed Lisa for letting Quentin "get away with murder." Lisa blamed Bob for poisoning the office with a "black cloud." Still, fed up, they knew it was important to band together and act. They confronted Quentin about his addiction and demanded he go to rehab. If he refused, they were prepared to dissolve the partnership, at a great loss even, and leave Quentin to fend for himself. If he agreed, they were prepared to pay for half of the rehab cost out of their own pocket. Relieved to have such a seemingly clear way out of the current crisis, Quentin agreed.

For a short time after returning from rehab, Quentin showed glimpses of his old self. But soon, though drug free, he reverted to all his unacceptable behaviors. He was now the painkiller version of a dry drunk, and it became clear that his accident and subsequent troubles hadn't created emotional problems but instead had brought preexisting ones to the surface.

By this time, Abby had begun working after school as a part-time receptionist at the office. This was supposed to provide some real-world responsibility for her, along with savings for college. She craved the money but burned through all of it almost instantly with her boyfriend, Ike. Feeling sorry for Quentin, she often covered for his mistakes, smoothed over the feathers he ruffled, and took his side whenever possible to get under her parents' skin.

THE FAMILY DYNAMIC

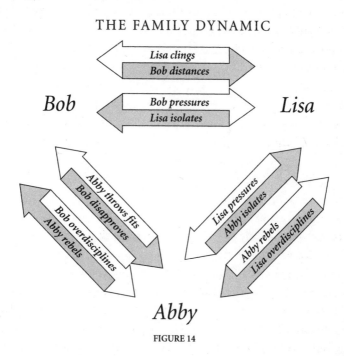

FIGURE 14

Meanwhile, at school Abby kept up a 4.0 average without even trying. She had her heart set on attending an Ivy League university and didn't worry about saving any of her own money because of a robust college fund her parents had started even before she was born. But now that fund was in jeopardy. If Lisa and Bob couldn't salvage their partnership with Quentin or receive a decent settlement, they'd have to draw down Abby's fund while starting all over.

When Lisa and Bob told Abby about this, she went berserk. She claimed that they were scapegoating Quentin and lying about their financial woes. She accused them of trying to get back at her because she didn't follow their rules and instead hung out with a guy who loved her like they never did. One night, when Lisa and Bob were asleep, Abby ran away to Ike's dingy studio apartment in the worst part of town.

She stopped going to school and wouldn't return any calls or reveal her whereabouts. The only communication Lisa and Bob received from Abby was a single text message letting them know she was safe.

As the weeks dragged on with no end to the crisis, Lisa neared a breakdown. She read about a weekend workshop of mine nearby, passed the information to Bob, and asked him if he'd come. He said they couldn't afford it, and besides, they needed practical solutions more than some "New Age crap." Lisa registered at the last minute anyway and showed up without him.

During the workshop, Lisa shared most of the story I've outlined here. Once familiar with the principles and practices of emotional connection, she wanted to know how it could be used to help improve things with Bob and Abby. The first essential component, I suggested, was to take complete responsibility for her own emotions. With Bob, that meant explaining to him exactly why and how her response to abandonment and inundation usually took place. In offering this explanation, it was crucial to stick to the past, a.k.a. the button, and not to focus on any of Bob's inciting behaviors. She might tell him, for instance, that whenever she perceives the threat of abandonment, her automatic resistance to it manifests as clinginess. Aware now that this was an old, unhelpful strategy, she could pledge her willingness to leave it behind in favor of feeling the abandonment directly.

This would simply set the stage, I told Lisa, and wouldn't mean much to Bob without seeing the process in action. That's why the second essential component was to communicate in real time whenever this cycle was taking place. For this, Lisa would need to stay attentive to her body, looking for the rapid heartbeat and rising shoulders that we'd earlier determined were her physical signs of contraction. Once she was aware a contraction had occurred, she could then describe it matter-of-factly to Bob, like an internal weather report.

Such a report would sound something like this: "Hold on a second, Bob. I just want to let you know that my heart is pounding, and my shoulders are tight. Let's pause the discussion for a few minutes to make sure things don't escalate."

The third essential component for Lisa was to perform the 2 X 2 process on her own, away from Bob, until reaching an expanded state. Usually, she could expect this to take anywhere from a couple of minutes to a half hour. Once complete, the last essential component was for Lisa to return to the previous conversation in the calmer, clearer condition that's the hallmark of expansion.

In this case Lisa would no longer be reactive. She'd be the one running the show instead of her resistance. She could talk about what was most important to her and even let her core emotions show without needing anything more from Bob than a sympathetic ear. I promised Lisa that if Bob saw this happen a few times and felt the resulting absence of pressure and demands, it would really register. There were no guarantees how he'd react, but without Lisa in her prior role, it would be impossible for their typical escalation to take place.

Key Refinement

DROP THE ROPE

When two people are in resistance, it's like a tug-of-war on top of a runaway train. The longer it lasts, the more dangerous it becomes and the harder it is to stop. Plus, no one can ever really win. Each seeming victory only makes the next go-round more difficult. Even people who seemingly refrain from fighting out loud inevitably find ways to yank the rope just as hard as the shrillest screamers.

But as soon as one person drops the rope, everything comes to a screeching halt. This simple act can often save an entire relationship, even if the other person doesn't yet have the will or skill to respond in kind. It's no easy task, however, because the momentum of that runaway train is often overwhelming. Just as any type of emotional connection requires physical awareness to proceed, so does dropping the rope. Yet once that awareness is present, anyone can do it. Here, simplified, are the steps I outlined for Lisa:

1. Recognize you're contracted.

2. Report the contraction to the other person as physical sensation only.

3. Pause the discussion and separate.

4. 2 X 2 until expansion occurs.

5. Resume the discussion, resistance free.

Regarding step 3, many couples choose to have a preset amount of pause-and- separate time that either party can invoke when things get heated, such as a "fifteen-minute rule." When this type of agreement is in place, it needs to be nonnegotiable, meaning that challenging its invocation isn't allowed. Otherwise, the rule itself can become just another excuse to resume the tug-of-war. If the necessary amount of 2 X 2 is accomplished before the set time ends, it's still a good idea to wait the full duration before reconvening. This helps any lingering tension dissipate. If the set time isn't enough to complete the 2 X 2, then whoever needs an extension is responsible to check in and request it. Within reason, this request should be nonnegotiable too.

When one person drops the rope, it not only stops any argument but also provides a significant opportunity for the one still holding it. Hearing about the contraction of one's counterpart is an invitation to see if something similar is occurring within. Then, in the space that's created by the unilateral pause, there's an additional inducement to let the dust settle and see the whole episode more clearly. Of course this may not actually happen for the remaining rope holder, but there's not even a chance of it happening as long as the tug-of-war continues. Lisa and Bob could point to almost twenty years of marriage as proof of that.

Lisa went home from the workshop committed to give this all a try. Within just the first moments back, her chance came. Bob, it turned out, was resentful that she had gone and was also smarting from another run-in with Quentin. He greeted Lisa with the kind of frostiness that usually caused her to stage a demonstrative, clingy scene. Instead of picking up the rope, Lisa calmly explained what she had learned at the workshop and was eager to put into practice. Bob was skeptical, as expected, but softened a bit when not even a trace of drama ensued. As they remained drama free over the next few days, amid lots of opportunities for their usual tug-of-war, Bob started to take real notice. Once, to Lisa's surprise, it was Bob who invoked the fifteen-minute rule that she'd introduced.

But then Bob pushed one of Lisa's buttons with what she considered brutal strength. Not surprisingly, it had to do with Abby. More important than the content of their tug-of-war in this instance was how it played out. First Lisa dropped the rope and asked for fifteen minutes. Then she needed another fifteen minutes, and another, and couldn't actually reach a modicum of expansion before bedtime. This left Bob to stew all night long, convinced that her drastically extended pause was just a fancy excuse to punish him with the same old disappearing act. By the time morning came, Bob was the dramatic one, hounding Lisa to "crawl out of her shell," cursing the workshop, and reeling in resistance to an intolerable turmoil that he claimed was all her fault.

Not sure of her own ability to handle such an uproar without reverting to old behaviors, Lisa left the house and reached me by cell phone. We began with the basic tools, 2 X 2-ing till she regained a state of expansion and felt confident in its durability. Then we talked briefly about what it means to create a positive boundary, and how to communicate safely and truthfully with one in place. The whole call took about twenty-five minutes. She apologized for "ruining" my morning, but in return I thanked her for having the courage to reach out. I reminded her how important it is to have a team in place for just such moments (see page 93), because there will always be situations when an emotional storm can't be fully weathered alone.

Key Refinement

POSITIVE BOUNDARIES

Most of the time, when experts talk about boundaries, it's from the standpoint of protection. Good boundaries are meant to provide a healthy way for everyone to keep their own "bad stuff" to themselves and especially to avoid soaking up more bad stuff from others. Often such boundaries are necessary and helpful, but they quickly become tricky for people practicing emotional connection. When erecting and maintaining a boundary is primarily a defensive act, this well-intentioned strategy actually promotes contraction. We become tight, suspicious, and in the process forfeit the pleasures and benefits of expansion. Luckily, there's an alternative.

A positive boundary is actually born of expansion. To create one, we connect to the state of well-being within ourselves and imagine it extending beyond the physical body in every direction. Surrounded by this cocoon of expansion, we're able to remain open but also safe. The same kind of comments and behaviors that usually push our buttons to the point of reactivity now seem no match for our good spirits. It's as if they make just a slight dent in our positive boundary and then fall away without even reaching us.

POSITIVE BOUNDARIES

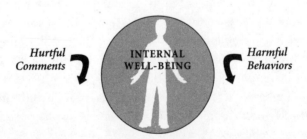

Hurtful Comments — INTERNAL WELL-BEING — *Harmful Behaviors*

Positive boundaries allow us to remain protected while still feeling good. Plus, our reactivity diminishes.

FIGURE 15

If this sounds too good to be true or as if it is some kind of self-delusion, try it a few times and see what happens. Most people report that it provides the greatest benefit at the riskiest times, such as holiday gatherings with family or fractious staff meetings. I recommended a positive boundary for Lisa because she was facing precisely the kind of situation that called upon all her reserves of forbearance. While it wouldn't serve her to remain totally undefended, she absolutely couldn't afford to shut down.

When Lisa returned home, she found Bob still stewing over her abrupt departure. He resumed his harangue without missing a beat and with greater intensity. But Lisa had already cultivated a positive boundary, and this succeeded at preventing Bob's barbs from penetrating hurtfully. Aided by the expansion her boundary had safeguarded, Lisa calmly told Bob that it was okay for him to share his feelings with her, but that if they were to remain in conversation he had to do so in a respectful way. Grudgingly, he agreed and first wanted to hear what *she* had to say.

Happy to oblige, Lisa told Bob that they both deserved a family environment in which no one was to blame for anyone else's feelings. And Abby did too. Lisa said she understood that her need for more distance after their last bout was painful to Bob, but that it wasn't just the same old pattern. In fact, it was the opposite. This time, even though his words had sent her spiraling deeper than ever into old wounds, she refused to retaliate. Inside Lisa's "shell" she hadn't been punishing Bob or defending against him. Instead, she'd been doing her best to stay clear and connected, both to herself and to him. She reminded Bob that she was new at all this and somewhat shaky. That's why she had to leave and seek some outside counsel. Now, Lisa promised, she was ready and able to help increase the degree of safety and support available to them both. If Bob would join her, Lisa wanted to begin that effort by trying to understand his experience better than ever before.

Like most of us, one of Bob's deepest desires was to be heard and understood.

PRACTICAL TIP

Whether it's apparent or not, almost everyone
craves to be heard and understood. To increase
the likelihood that your own emotional reality will
be honored, make sure you return the favor.

He accepted Lisa's invitation and talked with rare, vulnerable candor about how these simultaneous crises of marriage, work, and family had worn him down. He spoke, haltingly, of his honest doubts that their marriage could be saved and that he had it in him to give it a real try. He appreciated Lisa's efforts but thought it might be too late.

Lisa listened. She listened with her whole mind and body, soaking up not just each of Bob's words but also the feelings that came with them. She fought off every impulse to respond or try to change his mind. She asked gentle questions to understand Bob better, while still focusing on maintaining complete empathetic resonance.

During this conversation, something inside Bob shifted. Even as he was voicing a willingness to let their marriage go, he was also experiencing something truly new and different. Lisa was connecting with him in a way she never had. He felt that she saw and accepted him from the inside out and was willing to focus on what he needed for as long as necessary. It's not an understatement to say that he'd been waiting his whole life to experience such heartfelt, attentive caring.

You might wonder why this was possible only now, not previously during all of Lisa and Bob's relationship, and not even during any of their counseling sessions. The answer, first touched upon in the key refinement called tactical empathy (page 132–134), is that emotional connection to oneself is a prerequisite for genuine connection to another. No counselor can ever teach people to empathize before they're ready and before they've released enough resistance to allow it. All the credit here goes to Lisa, who bravely squeezed every chance for self-transformation from the workshop and subsequent challenges at home. In so doing, she provided a great example of how, when just one person changes in a relationship, the whole relationship changes as well.

Such changes aren't predictable or, for that matter, always positive. Fortunately, though, Bob was ready to follow Lisa's example. He did so quietly at first, just letting their encounter have its full impact on him without any kind of protective distancing. Then a few days later he started asking Lisa questions about the workshop and soon wondered if it might be a good idea for him to attend one too.

Lisa was overjoyed at this development but played it cool. Since no nearby workshop was scheduled in the immediate future, she offered to re-create a version just for him. She made sure to provide lots of conceptual framework, recognizing that men respond to that especially well, but also to guide him through enough 2 X 2 sessions that he could grasp the process experientially and begin practicing on his own.

Bob's first aha came when he realized that 2 X 2-ing minus any accompaniment could feel just as good as when Lisa had fully empathized with him earlier. His second aha was a vision of how breaking out of the family's deeply ingrained pattern of resistance might lead not just to the renewal of their marriage, but also to Abby's return. Bob asked Lisa to spend an evening with him thinking up all the things they wanted to say to Abby but previously had been too wrapped up in the pattern to get across. They used "preemptive empathy," a tactic of their own devising, to highlight and then edit any thoughts, feelings, or ideas that would be likely to push Abby's buttons. They didn't want to gloss over any of their truths but rather to present them in the most receivable way.

This surge of hopeful, creative energy, which their mutual expansion brought forth, still left them with a thorny dilemma. If Abby wouldn't talk to them, how could they get her to hear anything? Solving this dilemma involved a little ingenuity and also Bob's love of technology. First, Bob recorded a video of himself and Lisa speaking directly to Abby. Then he uploaded the video to a private page on their chiropractic office Web site. Finally, the two of them left a loving message on Abby's cell phone with information on how to view the video. After that, all they could do was wait and see if Abby's curiosity was stronger than her anger.

For a whole week nothing happened. Then Abby and Ike had a big fight. When she told Ike that an out-of-state college was in her near future no matter what and that their relationship wasn't meant to last, he acted out his hurt by throwing bottles across the apartment. Abby ran out in a panic and ended up staying overnight with one of her girlfriends. Shaken, she suddenly felt much more like a needy child than an independent adult. It was then that she borrowed her friend's computer to watch Lisa and Bob's video.

What Abby saw really surprised her. It was as if her parents had become different people, taking complete responsibility for their own shortcomings and not blaming her for anything. At the same time, they spoke to her more like a peer than a child. The clincher came when they shared their longing to be good parents, the sting of failure that followed each of their botched attempts at discipline, and their commitment to learning new approaches that would work for all three of them. Hearing that, Abby made the long-awaited call and agreed to meet, with no strings attached, at a local diner.

At the diner, Lisa and Bob remained vulnerable. They also let Abby know that her college education was a real priority, even amid all their current financial worries. They went on to provide Abby with revealing details of the Quentin saga that she hadn't yet heard. In this regard, as well, they reported rather than blamed, making it clear that if the office partnership could be saved, there would definitely need to be a three-way process. Impressed, relieved more than anything, Abby agreed to put her parents "on probation" and come home.

Wisely, for a while, Bob and Lisa let Abby reacclimate without any family meetings or new protocols. Before they got around to all that, Abby came to them, not entirely trustful but still keen to find out what had led to their markedly different behavior. That gave Bob and Lisa the opening to talk about their histories of emotional resistance and what had begun happening for them as they learned to let go. They also talked about what they had unconsciously passed on to her and how difficult it must have been to shoulder that burden. Without pushing, Bob and Lisa made it clear that the same path of connection that was working for them was also available to her. She listened but kept her distance and didn't take the bait.

Key Refinement

CONTAINMENT

Regarding when to practice emotional connection with oneself, we've looked previously at three strategies: in the moment that feelings or contractions arise, "not now, later," and "a little now, a lot later." But when should we communicate with others about this process or ask them to communicate with us? The way we answer these questions often determines whether our personal progress creates *inter*personal benefit.

There aren't many helpful rules, aside from dropping the rope, about when precisely to share feelings. That's because every social situation is dynamic and unique. But one skill in particular provides the maximum amount of freedom and flexibility, and that's containment. By containment I mean the ability to connect to a powerful feeling and then hold off on sharing it until an appropriate moment occurs.

Like resistance, many emotions compel us to *do* something, and talking about them is the most common form of action. But often we're not truly ready to talk, and the resulting conversation can make things more confusing and stressful. And even if we are ready to talk, often our conversation partners aren't. Here, too, mistimed dialogue can trigger fresh, unnecessary upset. When Abby finally agreed to come home, Lisa and Bob were excited to pass on their newfound emotional understanding and collaborate on a way forward for their family. But they also sensed it was too soon and decided in favor of containment. Their choice not only yielded a successful outcome but also created space for Abby to become the conversation initiator, which in turn increased her investment in the whole undertaking.

PRACTICAL TIP

When containment is necessary, but seems intolerable, use the 2 X 2 process to take the sting out of it.

Attempts at containment, in actual practice, only work if we can tolerate the frustration and impatience that may stem from refraining to communicate. Since the best way to tolerate all emotions is to connect to them, a focused application of 2 X 2 on any such frustration and impatience will almost always do the trick. In addition, whenever we're able to ride those feelings toward a more expanded state, we're also better able to determine when it's finally time to stop containing and start communicating.*

Back at the office, Lisa and Bob attempted the same kind of rapprochement with Quentin that they had with Abby. They got nowhere. In recent days Quentin had become even more bitter than before, convinced that the office partnership should be dissolved as soon as possible. He offered Lisa and Bob terms that were insulting, outrageous, and entirely untenable.

Lisa and Bob were blindsided, thrust into a classic fight-flight-freeze response, and forgot all about positive boundaries. Bob wanted to fight. Lisa wanted to flee. Recognizing his own hostility and not wanting to say anything inflammatory, Bob decided to clam up. This left Lisa to continue the discussion, and when she did so, hesitantly, it led to her own aha. Amid the clamor of her thinking and speaking, Lisa found herself able to practice a basic form of 2 X 2. She realized that emotional connection doesn't need to happen all by itself, and can even take place during a heated conversation. As a result, her words lost most of their charge. She quickly grew calmer, clearer.

---

*Many people, as you may have noticed, actually need to practice less containment, not more, moving through fear to communicate their emotions rather than conceal them. For them the best approach—no surprise—is first to find the flinch and then proceed with the usual steps.

PRACTICAL TIP

Emotional connection doesn't need to remain
a stand-alone activity. With practice, you can
2 X 2 all but the most intense feelings right in
the midst of any other endeavor.

The more expert we become at emotional connection, the less we need to call a time out, whether for fifteen minutes or otherwise. Furthermore, practicing the process during conflict harmonizes all three parts of our triune brain. This ensures that we're expanded enough to stay safe, feel, and think all at once. Such a harmonized state is exactly what's necessary to resolve conflict fairly and humanely, if at all possible.

In this instance it wasn't possible. Despite Lisa's best efforts, Quentin remained icy and unmoved. Crushed but willing to take the hit in order to live a less stressful life, Bob and Lisa prepared to move on.

Then, late one night, Abby knocked tentatively on their bedroom door. She entered visibly upset, needing to free herself of a heavy burden. She told them how, months before, Quentin had become flustered when crossing her path unexpectedly on his way out of the storage room. Following a hunch, Abby investigated some slightly out-of-place files. She wasn't certain, but she feared that Quentin was altering charts to overcharge on a number of worker-compensation cases.

Lisa and Bob were shocked that Abby would have withheld this information for so long, but they once again practiced containment, bit their tongues, and thanked her for coming forward now. The next day they conducted their own investigation and learned that Abby's find was just the tip of the iceberg. Quentin had not only defrauded the government of thousands of dollars, but he'd also siphoned money from the two of them directly. Armed with this information, they confronted him at once.

Rather than respond to their charges, Quentin went on the offensive. He claimed to be "shocked" that they'd distrust him in such an unforgivable way. He felt "sorry" that they were so paranoid and fearful.

He recounted a litany of times over the years that he had excused their "immaturity and incompetence." He pronounced them "spiteful and ungrateful," reserving his harshest attack for Lisa, whom he branded "the worst kind of traitor" for pretending to be his loving confidant while secretly plotting to bring him down.

Once again, Lisa and Bob found themselves in fight-flight-freeze mode, yet this time much more briefly. Lisa, in particular, put all her new tools to work with rare speed and skill. Using 2 X 2 to penetrate her contraction, she encountered not just her usual abandonment but also guilt at having caused Quentin such pain. Lisa knew instantly that this guilt was misplaced and that she'd done nothing wrong, yet she surfed through it rather than talk herself out of it. For a few moments she felt very young and helpless but soon expanded back into full power and presence. Believe it or not, all this happened while Quentin was still venting. By the time he was finished, Lisa had erected a positive boundary to ward off further attacks and to keep from becoming equally vicious herself.

Now able to see the situation clearly, Lisa easily recognized Quentin's attempt to avoid accounting for his own actions. But beyond that she also grasped the enormity of his projection, realizing that virtually every one of his accusations could also be read as a self-indictment. So instead of responding to any of those accusations, Lisa explained that the current situation was neither personal nor emotional. It was strictly about dollars and cents, about evidence that Quentin needed to address immediately.

Quentin continued to rant for another five minutes, first ignoring Lisa entirely and then claiming he had all kinds of damning evidence of his own. Finally, Bob stepped in. Softly but forcefully, he offered Quentin a choice: make restitution to all parties and dissolve the business on equitable terms or else face a lawsuit and a visit from the IRS.

Faced with this ultimatum, Quentin stormed out. But by the next morning, after a torturous night alone, he e-mailed Lisa and Bob his acceptance of the first option. Within a few days the dissolution paperwork was drawn up and signed. Within a week after that Quentin was gone. So, too, was a seemingly intractable problem.

Key Refinement

SEEING THROUGH PROJECTION

Projection, defined in the broadest way, occurs when we view one social interaction as if it's another. In so doing, we misplace our thoughts, feelings, or interpretations about a first person upon a usually unsuspecting second person. We may inaccurately assign the harmful motives of one neighbor, for instance, to another who only means us well. Or we may mistakenly trust a backbiting coworker who truly does mean us harm. As these two examples illustrate, projections can be falsely positive or falsely negative. But either way they're false, skewing our perception of reality with an erroneous mental overlay.

Most often projection involves seeing relationships in the present through the filter of those from the past. Unconsciously, for example, we may respond to the actions of romantic partners as if they were our parents. Lisa and Bob, as we've seen, spent years projecting in this way. In addition we can project our undesirable impulses and behaviors onto others—this is the standard psychological definition—as was the case with Quentin when he wrongly accused Lisa and Bob of his own transgressions. Finally, though less common, we can project other people's internal drives onto ourselves. With so much projection and so many varieties, life can begin to seem like a hall of mirrors in which no understanding of our relationships is reliable. Indeed, there are many thinkers who believe this to be true, considering all assertions to the contrary as mere delusion. These thinkers maintain that every human lens is unavoidably distorted not just by personal viewpoint but also by gender, race, class, culture, and a host of other factors. We pretend that there's one true reality in any situation, the reasoning goes, when in fact there are just degrees of distortion.

Regardless of how we assess this argument, however, less distortion is still better than more, and that's where emotional connection comes in. A resisted emotion is almost always what gives rise to problematic projections, both positive and negative. In fact, one helpful aspect of projection is that it shows us on the outside what we haven't yet been able to connect to on the inside. In this way projection functions just like the destructive life patterns that we've discussed earlier.

Here are some examples that span the history of the social network we've been investigating. If Quentin hadn't buried his guilt about stealing from Lisa and Bob, he would have had no cause to project his own immoral acts onto them. If Lisa still weren't resisting old feelings of abandonment, she wouldn't have taken Bob's need for distance so personally. If Bob hadn't been carrying a backlog of emotional turmoil, he wouldn't have viewed Lisa's upsets as such a threat. If Abby were conscious of the pain her parents' disapproval had caused her, she wouldn't have needed to glom on to Ike as a seeming salvation.

While it's evident that emotional connection diminishes projection, hopefully at this point you don't need further motivation to practice it. What you likely need, however, is a way to know when you *are* unduly projecting so you can put your tools to use. Such clarity is especially hard to achieve because by its very nature projection is almost always unconscious.

Fortunately, the way to make projection conscious builds upon the awareness that by now you've begun to master. The first dependable indicator of serious projection is physical contraction. If your primitive brain is labeling any seemingly benign interpersonal encounter a threat, and causing you to contract as a result, it's usually because of a similar past encounter that went badly and hasn't yet been emotionally cleared.

Suppose you have a nice, new boss, for example, who comes to your cubicle to see how things are going. While greeting him politely, you also notice a powerful flinch in your gut, and a corresponding paranoia that he's there to find fault with your work. Without your contraction's tip-off that you're projecting about a previous boss, you might respond in a jittery, defensive way that would actually *create* suspicion. But now with recognition, you can stay calm and clear during the rest of the meeting. Later, when the time is right, you can also 2 X 2 whatever's left over from the earlier situation.

In reading this example, you might wonder how to tell the difference between a gut feeling caused by projection and one that's important to heed. What if this seemingly benevolent boss were actually untrustworthy and you were correctly picking up on that? In general, such accurate intuition, if you pay attention to it, heightens your awareness and makes you a more effective communicator. It comes, in other words, contraction free.

The second reliable indicator of serious projection is an excessive emotional response. What's considered excessive in any situation is, of course, extremely subjective. While it's easy for other people to critique your emotions in this regard, the most important judge is you. If you deem your emotional response out of synch with what's happening, and that evaluation persists beyond your initial hit, then projection is likely afoot, and it's a vital time to 2 X 2.

Suppose you meet a new romantic prospect, for instance, and you're convinced that he or she is "the one." Before the first date has even concluded, you find yourself secretly imagining the marriage and children to come. Your heart pounds, your whole body swoons like never before. It feels too good to be true and, unfortunately, it is. All crushes, alas, are projection. It's not the actual person we relate to during such a crush but rather our wish for who they were. Whether or not any relationship turns out to be a keeper, no romantic counterpart can ever live up to that wish. Hence, the inevitable comedown. Which is not to say that you shouldn't enjoy your crushes while they last, but instead that an understanding of projection allows you to see them, and feel them, for what they really are.

The third and final reliable indicator of serious projection is when a current situation keeps luring your attention unpleasantly to something that seems similar from the past. In this case it's your thinking rather than contracting that's illuminating the parallel. But as long as the parallel is irritating and persistent, the diagnosis and prescription are the same.

Speaking of diagnosis and prescription, to drive home this point, imagine that you avoid going to see your doctor unless it's an emergency. Something about that office just bugs you. Visits there beset you with memories of your old pediatrician, who saw you through a painful, life-threatening childhood illness. As long as you stay away from your current doctor because of this negative association, projection will preclude you from receiving the best possible medical care. But as soon as you connect to whatever emotions are left from those early days of illness, your resistance to them will no longer hold you hostage.

PRACTICAL TIP

There are three reliable indicators that you may be projecting in a given situation: 1) physical contraction; 2) an excessive reaction; 3) persistent thoughts about a similar event from the past.

Before leaving the topic of projection, it's important to address the issue of other people projecting onto you. When this happens, there's an equally reliable indicator. It draws, not surprisingly, from some of the same clues we've been identifying. If the people in question are emoting at a degree that seems too intense for the situation at hand or are drawing dubious parallels to other events, there's a good possibility that they're projecting. At this point, however, you need to test your hunch further by asking them about it calmly and directly.

If these people are willing to take your question seriously and spend some time investigating it, they're either not projecting or will soon deproject via this very inquiry. Rarely will people honestly explore their projective possibilities, then deny everything and blindly keep it up. On the other hand, if your question draws any kind of heated response at the moment it's asked or over time, the likelihood of projection is high.

As long as people continue to project severely onto you, there's little chance in any dispute of finding solid common ground. In a way, for those projecting, it's as if the actual you isn't even there. That's why I recommend, if at all possible, leaving the scene and creating enough of a break in the action for everyone's vision to clear. Sometimes, just as with dropping the rope, such a break is the last best hope for resolution.

Over the six months following Quentin's departure, Lisa and Bob completely remodeled the office, and without having to raid Abby's college fund. The office's dark cloud lifted, and it felt warm and nurturing there once more. As a result, the practice grew by 30 percent. Abby, meanwhile, broke up with Ike, re-enrolled in school, and went back to her old job. Quentin, it came out later, hit rock bottom and temporarily ended up in a supervised facility. There he joined an ongoing support group and finally began to address the root causes of his predicament.

During this same period, Lisa, Bob, and Abby entered family therapy. With emotional connection as their foundation, they inched their way toward healthier communication and a set of household policies that everyone could buy in to and respect. Abby, in particular, made real strides in getting to her emotional core. These gains, to be sure, came in fits and starts with no happily ever after. Yet still, according to all three of them, their relationships continued to improve.

The social network described in this chapter contained only five people, but every observation presented can be applied to a group of any size. Emotional resistance plays a similar role in human dynamics whether there are dozens, hundreds, or even millions of people involved.

It corrodes not just individuals and families but also businesses, institutions, communities, and even nations.

Emotional connection, likewise, functions without regard to number. In addition, all the key refinements in this book can drastically improve any ailing, misdirected, or underperforming group. When one person or more begins applying them, it unleashes the contagion factor described earlier. People become able to think and speak more clearly and therefore function more effectively because they're no longer wrapped up in the endless, toxic, futile attempt to avoid emotion. If enough members catch the bug, the overall group culture is bound to change as well.

All it takes to quash such group transformation, however, is just one resistant naysayer with enough power and influence. That's why collective intention is so important. The best groups don't only promote emotional connection, but they also embrace and champion it as a part of their very ethos. They make emotional connection so welcome and rewarding that even the most powerful resister doesn't stand a chance. Granted, in our current society such groups are few and far between. But if you're lucky enough to find one, you'll realize it almost right away. The difference, not surprisingly, is something you can really feel.

A THOUGHT
EXPERIMENT

AFTER COMING SO far together in our exploration of emotional connection and its many benefits, let's conclude with a thought experiment. Imagine, for the next few moments, a world in which feelings truly got their due. This would begin with our system of education. Along with the three R's, every elementary school student would also learn their 2 X 2s. They'd know where emotions arise in their bodies. They'd know how to ride those emotions, as if at an internal amusement park. They'd know how to report their sensations during the ride and their insights afterward. They'd recognize their contractions quickly—as well as those of others—and make sure to "Feel first, think later, and talk last."

To some extent, this world is dawning. In the last ten years a rapidly growing field has emerged called social and emotional learning, or SEL. Many elementary, middle, and secondary schools now include some form of SEL curriculum. What's unfortunate, however, is that a majority of these programs emphasize emotional regulation, meaning how to make sure children don't act out or otherwise let feelings get the best of them. Can you sense the subtle resistance in that articulation? It's as if, following so much progress, we still identify emotions as part of the problem rather than part of the solution.

In our imaginary world, by contrast, emotions would be considered a true gift. Feeling them fully would be considered acceptance of that gift, as well as the way to put it to maximum use. This doesn't mean worshiping emotions, of course, or in any other way upsetting the balance of our overall mental harmony. Instead, consistent application of the 2 X 2 process is what would *ensure* that harmony.

Teaching 2 X 2 to children, however, would just be one change in our imaginary world. All adults would be required to demonstrate emotional mastery too. They'd receive ample training and testing on the evolutionary path for getting unstuck. They'd undergo annual contraction screenings, which would allow them to catch and correct imbalances early. They'd make important decisions, both personal and professional, only after correcting for whatever emotional resistance may be present. When meeting for first dates and assessing compatibility, they'd no longer ask about astrological signs, but would instead inquire, "What three emotions are the most difficult for you to feel?"

Granted, the previous paragraph is tongue-in-cheek, but it points out how emotional connection belongs most where it seems to belong least. Speaking of which, I once had a client named Glen, who came to me with a rare concern. "I'm confused about the Middle East," he said. Glenn was raised by Orthodox Jewish parents who believed that Israel was always right and its Arab neighbors were always wrong. As a teenager, he lived in Jerusalem for a year, and his loyalty to the Jewish state grew even stronger. As an adult, Glen watched the escalating violence in the Middle East through the lens of his survival response, always defaulting to the fight reflex. But then a friend helped him see Israel's shadows and imperfections, as well as the great suffering inflicted on innocent Palestinian families by this seemingly endless conflict.

Now Glen didn't know which policies to support. Other people might view such faraway issues as just politics, but Glen felt them viscerally. Using 2 X 2 revealed the physical aspect of his confusion as a pressure in his shoulders as well as an "anxious guilty buzz" from not having a clear position. Further emotional connection helped Glen accept ambiguity and uncertainty as both political realities and internal feeling states. This led him to uncover a deep sadness about the Middle East that he'd been resisting his whole life. Allowing the sadness to surface and flow brought Glen a degree of peace. He saw that a peaceful state within allowed him to view events more clearly than a compulsion to take sides and assign blame. Soon afterward he moved to Israel permanently, and while still engaging passionately in political analysis and debate, he joined an NGO that provided joint educational opportunities for Israeli and Palestinian children.

Glen truly is a trailblazer. Addressing matters that seem mostly about opinion and judgment, he went beyond his neocortex to develop a nuanced, authentic point of view. This point of view then led him to a course of action that was imbued with positive energy. He learned how to feel good and do good, simultaneously, in perhaps the most challenging locale on earth.

Along those same lines, I've often wondered what would happen if world leaders employed 2 X 2 in their policymaking. So continuing with our thought experiment, let's imagine a new kind of diplomat. Let's make the diplomat a strong, stoic-seeming man, to emphasize how risky and mold breaking his approach would truly be.

Our diplomat would realize that wherever emotions are shunned or considered inappropriate, they rule most forcefully behind the scenes.

CORE CONCEPT

Wherever emotions are shunned or considered inappropriate, they rule most forcefully behind the scenes.

Therefore, when preparing for important talks with foreign dignitaries, he'd clear his message and style of all emotional resistance. He'd ask the same of his entire staff. Then, before any negotiation, he'd 2 X 2 to maximize his internal harmony and make sure no disconnected emotions influence the proceedings. Finally, he'd take a rare, almost unimaginable step. After greeting his fellow diplomat warmly, he'd offer a candid, transparent self-assessment:

"I'm aware that a dispute with my teenage son has left me angry this morning. This inner state might render me more frazzled and impatient than usual, so please keep that in mind. If you ever notice that my family issue seems to improperly influence our communication, just let me know and I'll take a break to get back on track."

Our diplomat would also encourage his counterpart to offer a similar self-assessment. He'd honor whatever information was provided and gauge his responses accordingly. If his fellow diplomat proved less skilled or willing regarding emotional connection, he'd use tactical empathy (see pages 132–134) and all other applicable key refinements to secure the best outcome. He'd do all this as if the fate of the world were at stake, which might actually be the case. An avid student of history, he theorizes that emotional resistance among powerful leaders has led whole nations to ruin, sparked avoidable wars, brought about massive environmental damage, and caused the needless death of untold millions.

Let's take our thought experiment one step further, imagining that this diplomat goes on to get elected president of the United States. Governing with the same approach he brought to negotiation, the new president would invite the whole country to perform an emotional audit (see page 134–136). He'd ask American citizens to explore the role that emotional resistance plays in our approach to national issues. Is it possible, for instance, that intolerance of vulnerability causes us to turn our backs on the poor? Is it possible that inability to feel deprivation fuels our drastic overconsumption? Is it possible that unwillingness to feel shame leads us to overlook torture?

In the current atmosphere, just whispering such questions would amount to political suicide. Many of us won't bear the scrutiny and uncertainty that an emotional audit requires. Instead we tend to choose leaders who excel at empty reassurances. But in the world of our imagining, with a citizenry schooled in emotional connection, this call for national introspection would come across as an inspiring challenge, like JFK's famous proclamation about the moon mission.

Our extraordinary president, however, wouldn't stop there. He'd implore all Americans to discover what keeps us so disengaged from democracy. Is it possible, for example, that voter turnout is so low because we can't stomach disappointment? Is it possible that special interests corrupt the system because we're too afraid to fight back? Is it possible that we rarely rally for causes anymore because of a coast-to-coast epidemic of numbness?

While the answers to such questions aren't simple or clear, one thing is. Emotional resistance plays a similar role on the national stage as it does within each and every one of us. It's widely believed, for example, that Hitler never would have risen to power had the German nation not experienced such humiliation following WWI. From our perspective, however, humiliation wasn't the problem. Instead, it was resistance to humiliation that led Germany to embrace such a horrific way out. Had the population been willing to practice emotional connection and restored itself to greater well-being, perhaps the Nazi message would have been rejected long before wreaking havoc. Just as any organization can begin to realize its full potential by adopting an emotion-friendly approach, so, too, can any society. No longer can it be argued that such an approach makes people soft. To the contrary, it's the royal road to wisdom.

Let's return one last time to our imaginary world and president. In order to guide us beyond the crises we currently face, the president would challenge us to revisit the core values of our founders: freedom, fairness, tolerance, opportunity. He'd ask us to look with unblinking courage at all the ways we fall short in ensuring those values to every American. He'd encourage us to 2 X 2 through our contractions at those shortcomings, to practice mental detachment with each justification that arises, and to feel the whole gamut of emotions that such imperfection elicits.

Our president would point no fingers. Rather, his supportive leadership would help us move beyond red states and blue states to fifty newly expanded states. This nationwide expansion would rejuvenate our can-do spirit, unleash our collective genius, and promote policies that are equitable and sustainable. There would still be conflicts, certainly, since conflicts are an inevitable part of growth. But with emotional resistance at an all-time low, most conflicts would remain honest and civil. Exceptions to this shift would be spotted quickly and resolved skillfully. The more connected we'd grow to ourselves, the more vigorously we'd look out for one another.

In bringing our thought experiment to a close, and this entire book as well, I'm wistful. There's a heaviness in my chest and a welling in my throat. I know, alas, that no such politician exists. I'm not expecting one anytime soon. I'm also aware, however, that most profound change begins at the grass roots. So I invite you to join me in spreading the seeds of emotional connection in this world, the real world, until "we the people" fulfill our promise.

LINGERING QUESTIONS

IN THE PRECEDING CHAPTERS I've addressed most of the common questions about emotional connection and how to practice it effectively. In this appendix I've gathered additional questions and answers from workshops, presentations, client sessions, and reader e-mails. Some of them help tease out further depth and nuance regarding the process and its refinements. Others provide an opportunity to touch on the kind of thorny, everyday situations that can stop practitioners in their tracks.

How do I apply emotional connection to ADHD?

ADHD is both a label and a stigma. It refers to a vast variety of difficulties in focusing attention and maintaining stillness. In addition to attempting to diagnose it medically, I recommend using the 2 X 2 process with done-deal delay (see page 106) to find out what happens if you stave off, ever so briefly, the impulse to shift out of a current situation. It's probable that remaining in the situation will bring up one or more challenging emotions that are calling for connection. From this perspective, ADHD-type symptoms are often indicators of emotional resistance. Once the resisted emotions are incrementally yet fully met, the indicators no longer remain.

It's also true, of course, that each of us functions best at our own natural speed. Some people are born flitters, while others are more deliberate. If you happen to run at an unusually high rpm, emotional connection is not a cure-all. Here, the solution often lies in finding appropriately matching environments and activities for your temperament. This approach, however, also requires emotional connection for maximum gain. Without it you have no reliable way to determine whether your selection of environments and activities is coming from resistance or acceptance (see "fork in the road," page 130–132). With it, expansion becomes your barometer.

If you have a speedy, distractable, or otherwise problematic type of focus, you'll also find that emotional connection helps expand your range of possible responses to frustrating stimuli and situations. It enables you to tolerate more and more internal upset without having to escape immediately or act impulsively. This expanded range, in turn, grants you the freedom to determine whether, and how, to meet uneasy situations. In most cases this eliminates the need for medication. When it doesn't, emotional connection works in tandem with medication to create a synergistic benefit.

This whole approach is about breaking through barriers to live your dreams. But I've never been able to figure out what my dream is. Does emotional connection help with that?

Almost always when people don't have any kind of dream at all, it's because of numbness. The 2 X 2 process definitely penetrates that numbness, as demonstrated by a thirty-three-year-old client of mine named Sonia, whose lack of a dream made her feel like a "freak of nature." Whenever Sonia thought about what she wanted, she came up with nothing and felt nothing. The 2 X 2 process quickly rendered her less numb, but at first this only revealed lots of previously blocked aches and pains. Then the aches and pains receded, and Sonia accessed a chronic, low-grade anxiety.

Sticking with the process, dropping beneath that anxiety, Sonia uncovered a childhood storehouse of helplessness. She was orphaned at an early age, and her adoptive parents overcompensated by sheltering her from the inevitable slings and arrows of life. After a few more sessions, Sonia's helplessness gave way to a surprising hunger for adventure. While previously a city girl through and through, she started to camp and backpack. Eventually she fell in love with white-water rafting and soon found her passion guiding excursions along the Colorado River.

While your own passage through numbness will undoubtedly be unique, virtually all such journeys lead to a newfound sense of purpose. Apart from that, but just as important, they also heighten enthusiasm for everyday life.

My teenagers tune me out. Will emotional connection get them to listen?

Teenagers, and all kids for that matter, are constantly testing the limits of their power and control. Tuning you out is one way to say, *"You're not the boss of me."* The problem is that you still are, at least in many respects. When your teens disobey or ignore you and you resist the emotions that result, they sense that resistance and respond with more of their own. This is the phenomenon that we first covered in drop the rope, on page 165. While dropping the rope is certainly a good approach to keep tensions between you and your teens from escalating, here's another possibility.

Schedule a period of alone time to find the flinch, cut to the chase, and weather the storm regarding this communication breakdown. When your teens don't listen to you, for example, it may bring up a worst-case scenario that you're a terrible parent, and the feeling involved with that assessment might that of being total failure (as happened with Lisa and Bob in chapter 12). Letting yourself feel that sense of total failure will prevent you from becoming an actual failure. That's because you'll no longer need to resist when your teens tune out. Then, in the relative expansion that results, you'll also be able to assess the best, most appropriate response.

Sometimes, with some kids, the most effective response is to share honestly and vulnerably about the storm you've recently weathered. You might say something direct and straightforward, such as, "I've come to notice that when I get into battles with you, it's because I hate feeling like a bad parent. That's my issue, not yours. So I've decided to stop resisting those emotions and just feel them. I hope that's going to make me a little less tense around you from now on."

Offering your teens a candid glimpse like this, into both your vulnerable emotions and a healthy response to them, can elicit a surprising degree of cooperation. For other kids the best approach is humor. When they can no longer get under your skin like before and realize that you're now "hip" to them, a light and funny touch can far outdo a heavy hand. Either way, no matter how your teens react, at least the previous deadlock will be broken.

In describing protective and core emotions, you mentioned moving through anger to more vulnerable feelings like hurt, loss, abandonment, and grief. Is it also possible to go the other way? In my case, it's easy to feel small and fragile, but much more challenging to access assertive emotions.

Assertive emotions like anger can definitely be core and are often obscured by the kind of fragile, protective emotions you've described. In these cases, seemingly authentic and vulnerable responses are actually a defense, an unconscious strategy to avoid deeply resisted feelings of aggression or power. When this occurs, fortunately the 2 X 2 process still takes you to the heart of the matter.

You've talked about how to determine the best choice of action by using the 2 X 2 process. But what if there's no good choice, as in most divorces when people have to decide whether to stay in a hopeless relationship or break up a family?

The role of emotional connection, as we've discussed, is to make sure our choices aren't unduly influenced by resistance. When they are, that's not wrong or bad. It just means we'll continue to encounter similar situations in the future. If you stay married out of resistance to the guilt of divorce, for example, you're still likely to find yourself guilty within the marriage. And if you leave your marriage to stop feeling the desperation it brings up, you're almost certainly going to attract new, desperation-inducing counterparts.

Emotional connection also helps us think clearly and creatively, which often leads to the emergence of previously unforeseen choices. Without the stress that comes with resistance, a person facing the end of a marriage might reach breakthroughs in counseling that enable recommitment. Or suddenly a trial separation might make the most sense.

What emotional connection can't do, of course, is magically transform a crisis in which all good options have been exhausted. However, it still allows us to make our choices authentically and peacefully, even amid all the pain and hardship. With a harmonized mind we come to see that the eventual outcome is not available to us yet. A divorce that is initially quite distressing to a child, for instance, may later turn out to have built character. Or it may have fostered greater closeness with one or even both parents. Realizing that such outcomes are mostly beyond our immediate control frees us to heed the deepest voices within. In my experience, this approach always leads to the most positive results.

Surprisingly, when all is said and done, the best choice is often none at all. Many times my clients insist, "I have to make my decision right now!" No matter the topic of their decision or the reason for their urgency, I usually suggest finding a way to postpone the moment of truth for a month, week, or even a day. Inevitably, something happens during that period that turns confusion to clarity.

PRACTICAL TIP

When you're still confused about an important choice after 2 X 2-ing fully, don't decide till the last possible moment. Most likely, with a little extra time, the answer will present itself.

Patience also plays a part when you know the right decision but you're not yet ready to make it. I had one client who took three years to file for divorce. All his friends and relatives were screaming at him to stop putting it off. At times he almost succumbed to their pressure, convinced that his delay was more about paralysis than wisdom. My job at those times was to highlight how emotional connection had already changed him profoundly in ways that his critics weren't willing or able to see. Finally, when he did file, there was no stress to it at all. The whole thing, in his words, "seemed to happen almost all by itself."

What am I supposed to do when weathering the storm really does feels like it'll kill me?

There are two kind of emotional resistance: hard and soft. The hard version occurs when for whatever reason it's not appropriate to open to your feelings fully. This might happen, for instance, when life demands that you focus elsewhere. Perhaps your child needs attention, or a deadline at work takes priority. Additionally, this hard version happens frequently in cases of serious emotional trauma that must be handled with great caution and professional assistance. In these cases, until your system is strong enough to handle the surges that emotional connection can bring, weathering the whole storm is definitely not advised.

The soft version of emotional resistance occurs when there's no legitimate reason not to connect, but your fear of the process gets in the way. You decide, "It'll just be too much," or, even more emphatically, "It'll kill me." When working with soft resistance, it's important to remember that no one really dies from emotion. Resistance to emotion, on the other hand, does create all kinds of health challenges. In our emotionally avoidant culture we choose the term "stress" to describe this, but most of the time that's just another word for the internal battle that resistance generates.

Discussing soft resistance always brings to mind a client of mine who was using the 2 X 2 process to quit smoking. Reporting her experience as withdrawal symptoms struck, she told me that her heart was pounding, her palms were sweating, and her stomach was all tied up in knots. I looked at her calmly and compassionately and wondered if she could just "be with" all of that. She looked back at me with narrowed eyes and asked, "For how long?"

Truthfully, there's only one answer to her question—for just this moment. In other words, when dealing with difficult experiences, it's often a great consolation that we only have to endure them one moment at a time. We never have to concern ourselves with the next week, day, hour, minute, or even second. Emotional connection only requires us to stay present to what's happening *right now.*

CORE CONCEPT

**You never have to stay present to any feeling
longer than just this very moment.**

When frustrated with painful emotion, we often have thoughts such as, *I can't deal with this heartache for even one more day.* But that kind of thought is about the future, not the present, and instead of having any impact on what will actually happen tomorrow, it only makes it more difficult to connect in this moment. If you find yourself hindered by thoughts about future emotion, approach them in the same way as analyzing, judging, assessing, and bargaining (see chapter 5). The key is not to fight them, but instead to note their presence dispassionately and then resume the 2 X 2 process as soon as possible.

Once you understand the difference between hard and soft resistance, the question still remains: without the occurrence of any telltale thoughts, how do I determine which is which? The simple method is to continue your application of the 2 X 2 process for about another minute. If your resistance is hard and therefore necessary, it will persist. At that point, stop the process with a recognition that now's not the time. If your resistance is soft and therefore unnecessary, it will melt away on its own and allow you to keep going.

DISTINGUISHING BETWEEN
HARD AND SOFT RESISTANCE

Resistance + 2 x 2 Process ————— = RESISTANCE *This is hard resistance and must be heeded.*	Resistance + 2 x 2 Process ————— = RELEASE *This is soft resistance and can be worked through.*

FIGURE 16

Finally, when working with soft resistance to unusually powerful emotions, it's important to keep in mind that you're only able to proceed successfully as fast as the slowest part of you can go.

PRACTICAL TIP

**You're only able to proceed successfully as fast
as the slowest part of you can go.**

If you go too fast, or push too hard, you'll find yourself in self-opposition (see page 107) and an inevitable pushback will result. You already have a number of tools to keep your connections at a sustainable, pushback free intensity and pace. These include pinpointing, cradling, and aligning yourself with the internal witness as Bryce did (see below). If employing all these tools still leaves you feeling overwhelmed, then it's definitely time to work with a skilled counselor.

What if a feeling always brings up hard resistance? Even with a counselor?

Another way to put this question is, "What if there's an emotion that I just can't or won't feel?" As for your unwillingness to feel an emotion, that's ultimately something that only you can address. When you're ready, you're ready, and attempting emotional connection even just one moment sooner will inevitably create pushback. So in this regard patience along with acceptance of your resistance provides the best way forward.

As for emotions that you can't feel even when applying all our key refinements, that happens most often due to a sense of inundation, meaning that the feeling seems to temporarily overpower your ability to witness it. I say "seems to" because in actuality that's an illusion. The best way I can exemplify this illusion is to share the story of Bryce, a forty-two-year-old from Vancouver, Canada. Bryce participated in an extramarital affair for three years. When the truth finally came out, it destroyed his family.

When we met, not surprisingly, Bryce was racked with guilt. He carried it with him everywhere, terrified, only able to connect to it in fits and starts. Over a number of sessions, Bryce allowed a little more unfiltered guilt to surge through. During our pivotal session, he reported that the guilt had become all-consuming and that every part of him was "on fire." I reminded Bryce that since he was aware of the guilt, witnessing and describing it, at least a thin shred of him remained separate, unembroiled. Grudgingly he confirmed this. Next, Bryce followed my suggestion to let that thin shred of awareness become much more microscopic and to cradle each and every newly arising sensation. Within a few minutes the guilt finally began to ease. In his mind's eye Bryce now glimpsed a dim light and had an inclination that at some point in the distant future he would once again be okay.

What Bryce's experience highlights is that your witnessing function never disappears, even for a split second. And as long as you're able to witness an emotion, you can also feel it. Therefore, whenever confronted by inundating emotions, temporarily pause the 2 X 2 process to reconnect with your inner witness first.

Often, it's just such inundating emotions that lead the way to our most valuable insights. Another client of mine, Donna, experienced this while on the other side of an affair. At first, when it came out that her husband had been unfaithful through their entire marriage, the feelings connected to this betrayal were too much. All she wanted to do was "shrivel up and disappear." Gently, I reminded Donna of the courageous African American women at a classic New Orleans funeral. These women trail the casket howling and wailing inconsolably. As a result they heal through their grief faster and fuller than anyone else.

A couple of months later, when Donna was ready to take on this emotional assignment, she reconnected to her inner witness and dove in. Her feelings ranged from rage and hatred to abject despair. But these feelings also brought her a fresh, expanded perspective. Without rushing or forcing the issue, Donna grew to recognize all the signs of marital distress that she had long ignored or denied. More important, she also recognized how remaining in an emotionally disconnected marriage had mirrored and served her own need to stay shut down. Without overcoming this emotional inundation, Donna never would have taken responsibility for her part in the relationship's shortcomings. She would have remained a victim, a questionable role model for her young daughter, instead of spending the next year cultivating a hard-won sense of vitality and independence.

I'm in sales, a field in which rejection is a constant source of frustration and burnout. How does emotional connection help when an unpleasant feeling is bound to return again and again?

To reprise an earlier answer, you never actually have to deal with rejection that hasn't happened yet. That's true whether the rejection eventually arrives in the next week, month, or year. You only have to deal with any rejection that may be arising right now, in this moment. Just that realization alone can seriously soften rejection's sting.

To reprise a main theme of this book, any emotion, rejection included, is a dynamic rather than fixed phenomenon. It's never the same from moment to moment or from situation to situation. Emotions only seem that way when approached either from a great distance or through the prism of resistance. When emotions are experienced with sustained bodily attention, both slow and microscopic, they reveal themselves as a rapidly shifting array of sensations flowing toward release.

Now, what does all that have to do with your job in sales? It means that from now on you no longer have to experience rejection per se. Sometimes you might have a burning feeling in your belly, a clammy flush to your cheeks, an inward pull of your torso, or a myriad of other painful but completely temporary sensations. If you're willing and able to meet these sensations with the 2 X 2 process, along with its refinements, they will all quickly pass away, leaving you expanded and refreshed for your next client call. And if you meet any associated negative thoughts with the practice of mental detachment, these, too, will depart harmlessly and posthaste.

I hope you'll take this depiction with a healthy dose of skepticism yet at the same time remain open enough to experiment. Usually it takes about a week of consistent, diligently applied 2 X 2 for the full benefit to take effect. You have absolutely nothing to lose in the effort and a major increase in job satisfaction to gain.

Sometimes, when I'm upset, I talk to the hurting part of me with the wiser part of me. I send myself "good parent messages" that everything is going to be okay, and this usually calms me down. Do you agree with this approach? Does it conflict in any way with emotional connection?

When discussing different approaches to well-being, my first advice is always "Whatever works." You mention that you're able to achieve a calming effect from this practice, and that's important. You also have firsthand experience of this benefit, which is much better than just believing it because you read about it in a book, whether mine or anyone else's.

Still, ever so subtly, you may be telling the upset part of yourself that it *needs* to calm down and that therefore there's something wrong with its current experience. This creates the risk of self-opposition and the pushback that inevitably results. That's why I prefer the less dialogue-focused method of cradling. It sends a message to our upset that is completely spacious and accepting. In light of this I'd suggest that you experiment with cradling during your next few upsets and see what happens. If for whatever reason you decide to return to your previous approach, just keep an eye out for any self-opposition. As long as there's none present, you have nothing to worry about.

In my circles there's a strong belief that what you focus on grows. So why would I want to bring what you call "exquisite attention" to my unpleasant feelings? Shouldn't I focus instead on uplifting emotions?

This view (first addressed in "Yeah, but" #5, on page 25) keeps growing in popularity. But unless fully understood, it's confusing and unhelpful. To focus on uplifting emotions is, indeed, a great practice for increased happiness and success. This is only true, however, if you're not already feeling something less pleasant. Attempting to change your feelings because you deem one kind better than another is bound to fail, creating substantial pushback and a high potential for self-sabotage.

Here's why: unpleasant emotions remain harmfully in your body until felt and released via the 2 X 2 process or something similar. The longer the emotions remain, the more intense they become, requiring greater degrees of resistance to keep them in check, which in turn saps the very positive energy that you're trying to increase. Therefore, you can't wish unpleasant emotions away. Nor can you ignore them away. Attempting to transform unpleasant emotions by focusing on their opposite is like building your dream house on a volcano. My advice in this regard is always plain and simple: When unpleasant emotions are present, begin by feeling your way to expansion. Then, and only then, focus your attention on what inspires you. Proceeding in this order ensures that you'll achieve maximum benefit for your efforts.

I understand the idea that I can't bypass my bad feelings by trying to feel better ones, but aren't there just times when enough is enough? What if I'm in a foul mood, and thirty minutes on a treadmill is all it would take to set me right? Wouldn't hanging out in my misery at that point just be a kind of masochism?

For most people, hanging out in their misery involves a self-perpetuating feedback loop between thoughts and feelings. Rather than practicing mental detachment, they either align with their negative thoughts or fight them. This, you're absolutely correct, keeps the whole painful experience locked unnecessarily in place. Both the unwanted thoughts and feelings just keep on coming, sometimes repeating themselves ad nauseum and other times arriving in new, original variations of the same old torment. It's possible to remain in this state not just for hours or days but even a whole lifetime.

Emotional connection, by contrast, clears this cycle at its source. You may recall the way that happened for Tom, Jordan, and Barbara in chapter 4. It will happen for you in the same way, as long as your 2 X 2-ing is accompanied by consistent mental detachment.

On the other hand, it's important to note that some bad moods aren't about emotional repression at all. They may be hormonal or otherwise randomly induced by an imperfectly functioning organism. In these cases—you're right—all the 2 X 2 in the world isn't likely to produce more than minimal expansion. Plus, the emotions produced at such times are far less trustworthy than usual.

Therefore, if you become aware that your emotional connection is either abnormally intense or negative, pause momentarily and perform a mood scan. Does everything you consider seem to have a similar cast? Has this been occurring for more than an hour? If so, take the currently arising emotions with a grain of salt. And by all means, as you've suggested, shift activities and see what happens. Sometimes vigorous exercise does do the trick, providing a kind of system reset. At other times sleep leads to the same result, as can complete concentration on something outside yourself. Whichever you choose, just make sure you're also accepting the bad mood in the same way you would an individual emotion. Resisting a bad mood, inevitably, makes it last longer and feel much worse.

When I open enough to connect to my own emotions, I start feeling other people's emotions as well. This is usually very painful and almost always overwhelming. Is there anything I can do to stop it?

Emotions are indeed contagious. You can catch them through a prevailing social atmosphere (as described in chapter 13), or merely one-on-one. For those of us who are particularly sensitive to emotions, becoming overwhelmed is a common problem. I've had a lot of clients who actually choose to limit their contact with others to mitigate this hazard.

Fortunately, however, there are two easier and less restrictive ways to stay just as safe. The first way is to erect a positive boundary (see page 167). Such a boundary works to not only ward off people's hurtful comments and behaviors as described previously but also to keep their emotions at a manageable distance. The second way to stay safe is especially recommended for those who'd rather steer clear of extra boundaries but still avoid taking on any more emotion than necessary. It entails practicing the 2 X 2 process for every feeling, regardless of its origin, while imagining that your body is a porous screen door. Those emotions that initially arise inside of you will now still release in the usual way. Those emotions that arise outside of you will pass through the screen door quickly and easily and without much need for attention.

PRACTICAL TIP

When you're not sure if certain emotions "belong" to you or those nearby, imagine that your body is a screen door. Emotions that flow through the door like a breeze aren't of concern. Those that stick, on the other hand, are yours to feel.

Every once in a while an emotion from outside of you will stick to your visualized screen door. Whenever this happens, the emotion is yours to feel. That's because this external emotion has resonated with a parallel internal emotion and dislodged it, so to speak, from the protective custody of your resistance. In that sense, it's a blessing. The external emotion has made you aware of resistance that was previously unconscious. Now, if you're willing to 2 X 2, it's usually no more difficult to clear this inside-outside combo than any ordinary personal emotion.

My own sensitivity isn't about experiencing other people's passing emotions. Instead, I feel like I've been taken over by my father's entire emotional makeup. I literally feel his responses inside me more powerfully than my own. Whenever I try to relax, for example, his voice booms in my mind, "You can play when you finish your work, and your work is never done." So I'm wondering, is there a way to perform an emotional exorcism?

Your question is about the emotional legacy that parents hand down to children, which we first explored in chapter 13. It reminds me of a client from many years ago, Carrie, who was bright, beautiful, and psychologically savvy but at thirty-three had never been in a long-term relationship. Here's how she described it: "I have an overpowering version of my mother inside of me and she's convinced that I don't deserve to be happy and am always wrong. As a result I never stand up for myself. I always pick the most messed-up guys. I find a way to sabotage even bad relationships." The tone in Carrie's voice made it clear she was fighting an internal civil war and losing badly. Such a civil war thrives upon an either/or orientation. To keep it going, we must remain deeply contracted, with only enough room at any time for just one side to hold the battlefield. So I worked with Carrie on a both/and approach, which in this case meant meeting the version of her mother with absolutely no resistance. It meant, instead, connecting with the emotions that had split off into this mother persona and were fueling Carrie's entire conflict.

It took many false starts and about a half hour for Carrie to 2 X 2 with her avowed enemy, but once in full flow, she unleashed a flood of unworthiness. This unworthiness had been passed from one generation to the next. Fair or not, it belonged to Carrie now. To end both the war and the legacy, in an ironic twist Carrie needed to cradle her own mother. It took a few additional sessions and a lot of repeating as necessary on her own, but within about a year Carrie felt mostly at peace. Within another year came a healthy, durable relationship.

PRACTICAL TIP

The best way to heal harmful versions of parents or others who live inside you is to cradle the feelings they induce.

What's required in your case rather than an "exorcism" is an internal reunion similar to the one Carrie experienced. This means embracing the emotional reality of your father as it lives within you fully enough to feel all that he couldn't. The resulting healing will free you from your emotional possession, reconnect you with your own authentic inner voice, and ensure that you pass on a healthier legacy.

You've mentioned "proportional response" (see page 152) as a way to feel only what's safe and necessary in a given situation. Is there also such a thing as "proportional vulnerability"? Sometimes staying open doesn't really seem appropriate for me, especially at work. And in relationships I notice that I do better sharing my emotions a little, but not too much. Do you see this the same way?

Proportional vulnerability makes perfect sense. My one caveat is that you can only ascertain the best degree of vulnerability to match each situation when you're in an expanded state. Therefore, when making your assessment, always 2 X 2 first and fully.

Your focus is on the way we resist our own emotions. But what I resist most is the emotions of others, and especially their judgments. I devise elaborate strategies to make people love and appreciate me and to avoid their criticism and rebuke. How can I stop doing that?

The only reason you ever need other people to feel a certain way about you is to change the way *you* feel about you. When you strategize so much to win their love, it's a reflection of how unloved and/or unlovable you actually feel. It's even more reflective of your resistance to those feelings. If the feelings weren't intolerable to you, there would be no reason to seek their opposite. The same is true about strategies to avoid criticism.

Remember: most of the time we're either running toward a feeling or away from one. It's probably even more accurate to say that we're doing both at the same time. In your case this is certainly true. But so far you've placed the majority of your attention on the role others play in that process. This can work but only to a point, since the people in our lives have an uncanny knack for not following the script! So I suggest that you experiment with cutting out the middleman and going straight to the source of your greatest influence and impact—yourself. Use the 2 X 2 process to release your resistance and weather the storm of those difficult feelings that you've been forever desperate to avoid. Once the storm clears, you'll feel expanded and free no matter what anyone else has to say about it.

I don't really mind when other people judge me. That's probably because I'm pretty judgmental myself. Is that so bad, especially if it's just the truth about how I feel?

From my perspective you're free to judge all you like, but it's important to recognize the emotional underpinnings of judgment as well as its emotional consequences. Generally, judgment is about determining what's good and bad, right and wrong. In practice, however, we focus primarily on the bad and wrong. Judgment, therefore, tends to be critical. That's just as true about self-judgment as it is about the type you're describing. Either way, judgment is a resistance mine-field. It's often a strategy to avoid vulnerable feelings rather than an accurate description of our true viewpoint. As a result, maximum well-being requires that we determine the type of judgment that's afoot. To do so, apply the 2 X 2 process in regard to your feelings about any person or issue that you're judging. Then, notice whether the judgment remains once you reach an expanded state. If so, you can rest assured that it's not causing you any emotional detriment.

CORE CONCEPT

Judgment without resistance becomes discernment, and in the process promotes expansion.

Most of the time, though, you'll discover that judgment and expansion are incompatible. That's because judgmental thoughts tend to have a smug or self-righteous quality. While such qualities may provide brief and superficial satisfaction, overall they leave us brittle, tense, and stuck. Still, in the service of expansion, there's no need to surrender our opinions and values. Instead, all that's required is that we refresh them often with emotional connection. Then, in the aftermath, we submit those views to the scrutiny of a newly harmonized mind. What happens as a result is that most judgment loses its resistant bite while maintaining its power and specificity. In this way judgment becomes *discernment*, which is not only compatible with expansion but also promotes it.

I have a big "Yeah, but" to the previous answer. There are lots of things in life that are worthy of condemnation—like child abuse, for example—and if remaining brittle and tense is the price I have to pay to sustain my condemnation, so be it. I'm not so interested in my own happiness if it means letting evil people off the hook.

Your question contains a common either/or scenario, assuming that to hold on to your condemnation of evil, you must feel bad. I invite you to consider the both/and scenario—that you can fight for a just world *and* feel uplifted by your efforts. In fact, I maintain that you'll become a much more effective activist for change if you approach the issues involved from an expansive, discerning orientation. The evils of the world, no doubt, will follow their own course completely independent of how open or closed you feel. When holding on to your resistant judgments of other people, it's you who pays the price for their actions, not them.

You've mentioned a few times that emotional resistance takes place not just with individuals and groups but even at the national level. Can you be more specific about that?

The most illustrative answer to this question involves patriotic pride, the idea that one's own country is better than all the others. In America this view is quite prevalent. Many people who have never even set foot on foreign soil are convinced that every other nation is less creative, less free, and an overall worse place to live. What's of interest to us here is not whether that's actually true or can even be measured, but rather the way people cling to this viewpoint reflexively and become uninterested in debate or new information.

Reflexive viewpoints are a reliable sign of resistance, both at the personal and social levels. Here, there seems to be a need for Americans to feel that they are the "best." This points to the inability to feel inferior or even just equal to the other nations of the world. Like all types of emotional resistance, it comes at great cost. Both citizens and officials alike routinely dismiss international surveys that rank America low on indexes for things like academic achievement and quality of life. Just this week, as I've been mulling over our unconscious resistance in this regard, UNICEF released a study that ranks the United States at the bottom of twenty-one wealthy countries in overall child welfare. Whenever something like this happens, pundits are quick to either attack a study's conclusions or sound a panicky state of alarm.

If freed from resistance to feelings of equality and inferiority, we'd probably chart a middle course, welcoming such a study as an opportunity to take a good look at ourselves. We might still evaluate the study for accuracy, but we'd also immediately address whatever bona fide shortcomings in our society it reveals. Further, we might organize missions of inquiry to the highest-ranking countries to discover successful strategies of theirs that can be replicated here. Some of these responses do occur in academic institutions, but overall we tend to be allergic to them. Imagine the outcry if the president of the United States went on television and said that we have a lot to learn from the Czech Republic or the Scandinavian countries. What if he invited the leaders in child welfare from these countries to come to America, study our weaknesses, and offer advice for improvement? Almost certainly, that president's approval rating would instantly plummet.

To be clear, my point is not about the relative merits of countries or studies. Instead, I want to draw attention to the way any population's unwillingness to feel humble and vulnerable about itself will severely limit opportunities for growth and improvement. This principle also works in reverse. Populations that are unwilling to feel positive and powerful about themselves will also limit their potential for growth and improvement. Therefore, only a nation that does not need to feel or deny any particular emotion is completely free to chart its own expansive destiny.

When telling Kenneth's story (see pages 143–145), you described how the 2 X 2 process helps reveal the degree to which physical complaints are actually somaticized emotion. I'm wondering if the 2 X 2 process can help alleviate pain, period, regardless of its source?

When viewed slowly and microscopically, pain of any type, just like emotion, is a series of rapidly changing sensations. We applied this recognition a few questions ago when looking at my client's withdrawal symptoms, but now let's broaden our consideration. Take a headache, for example. Technically, there's no such thing. During the 2 X 2 process, a headache might express itself as pulsing at the temples, then a gripping sensation at the back of the neck, then pressure along the top of the scalp, then no sensation at all for a split second, and then pulsing once again. Approaching a headache with this kind of attention creates a gentle, spacious internal environment. Usually, this is just what a headache needs to lessen considerably, and even disappear.

The same is true for any type of chronic pain. Speaking as someone who's lived with a debilitating ailment for two decades, I can attest that the word "chronic" is more conceptual than experiential. Even my most persistent symptoms arrive in new and different forms with every passing moment.

PRACTICAL TIP

Chronic pain is a concept. The experience of any pain, moment by moment, is always changing.

And whenever I greet these symptoms with 2 X 2, the actual pain always decreases. Plus, in those rare instances when I choose to take medication for my condition, the dulled symptoms that follow still respond best to this approach.

I've been experimenting with a both/and orientation to my inner conflicts, and it's not pretty. Almost every time I have to do something—like study, go to work, exercise—there's another part of me that rears up and says, "No! I don't wanna!" How am I supposed to handle that?

Inside most of us there's a terrible two-year-old just like the one you describe. Of course I don't mean this literally, but much of our everyday resistance definitely bears a whiny, babyish tone. The problem only starts, however, when we decide that there's something wrong with this response. It's then that the test of wills begins, and as any parent knows, a two-year-old can take you to the mat. Yet while our whiny resistance seems to stand in the way of necessary activities, what it usually wants is just to stomp around and complain. If we let it, the resistance soon settles, and we're able to go about our business.

Personally, I experience such an "I don't wanna!" response before each and every speech on my schedule. It arrives without fail the night before, when suddenly all I can think about is room service and bad TV. Sometimes I indulge those desires in moderation, and sometimes I don't. No matter what, though, I offer my stompy resistance a genuinely warm welcome. I hear and acknowledge its contrary desires without condescending or editorializing. I've seen time and again how it's my acceptance, more than any back talk or indulgence, that unfailingly silences the whine.

My husband and I work together. He's very bossy and won't collaborate in a way that feels good to me. After all these years I know he's not going to change. And I know I'm not going to get a divorce, quit the business, or force him out. But I'm also tired of fighting about it, of going into my whole "I can't take this anymore!" routine. When I do the 2 X 2 process, I go from angry to sad and then just basically stay that way. Is there anything more I can get out of it?

This is an important question, because so many people find themselves in situations that aren't realistically changeable. Clearly, you've already done the initial work of following your emotions from protective to core. The place you're now stuck, it seems, is one of the most common.

The best way to describe this sticking place is a slightly expansive plateau. In your case, the experience of sadness is authentic and flowing enough that you've been willing to pause there and catch your breath, so to speak. At the same time, however, you may also have slacked off a bit with your attention and lapsed into a little judging and bargaining. If so, the judging may have shown up in thoughts like, *It's not okay with me to be so sad all the time.* The bargaining might have shown up in thoughts like, *I'll agree to keep going with all this on the condition that I get to feel something different.* The irony for all of us who arrive at this point is that we do get to feel something different eventually but only if we can cease judging and bargaining.

From now on, if any such judging and bargaining occurs, accept it calmly with no added resistance and turn your attention directly to the physical center of the sadness. Through this recommitment to the process, you'll find, as we've been touching upon repeatedly, that the sadness will present itself as a lively, ever-transforming array of sensations. Attending to this array will eventually bring you greater peace and joy. This peace and joy may supplant your sadness or paradoxically occur right along with it. In other words, proficiency at emotional connection makes it possible to feel expanded, sad, and joyful nearly all at once. Such multiresonant states arise when your *yes!* to the moment at hand is both passionate and unequivocal.

I'm not more sensitive than the next person, but I do tend to take things very personally. If the gas-station attendant scowls at me, for example, I can't get it out of my head for hours. Intellectually I know it's not about me. I mean, he's probably just having a bad day or something. But that doesn't keep me from obsessing about it. Can I do anything about this?

The simple way not to take things personally is to recognize that emotions are mostly spontaneous, unavoidable responses to your surrounding environment. A sunset might make you feel peaceful, a storm might make you feel afraid, and a rude clerk might make you feel irritated. It seems like the clerk is doing something *to* you, but in essence he's just another part of the landscape. If you take his scowl personally, it's because analyzing and judging have blocked your emotional flow. Instead of just registering the arising emotion and allowing it to pass away, you get stuck wondering *why* this experience has happened and determining all the things that are *wrong* with it.

When analyzing and judging continue obsessively, it's because your reasoning brain (neocortex) and your feeling brain (limbic system) are locked in a stalemate. Your reasoning brain thinks that if it can solve the current "problem" or accurately assign blame, then all will be well. In the heat of the moment it forgets our motto: "Feel first, think later." Out of order and misdirected, it's blind to its own true motive—get rid of the emotion. The more it attempts to banish the emotion, the stronger the emotion fights back. This stalemate inevitably persists, growing ever more painful, until you become aware of what's happening and intervene.

Here's how: As soon as you notice that anything from your external environment has provoked a personal response, begin 2 X 2 immediately. Keep surfing, letting all analysis and judgment drift through you like internal clouds. Soon the clouds will clear, and so will the previously blocked emotions. The why of it all won't matter in the same way, and neither will blame. And if there is indeed something about the situation that bears nonresistant examination, you'll now truly be up to the task.

In case this seems too easy, consider the example of my client Jerry. A high-school track coach, Jerry worked daily with unappreciative, disrespectful athletes. Their insolence got under his skin to the point that he considered quitting. He just couldn't understand why today's kids are so entitled (analyzing), and he really thought it was his job to set them straight (judging). During a brief round of 2 X 2, Jerry broke through his fierce resistance and encountered a profound sense of disappointment. This disappointment sat in the center of his chest and burned like hot coal. After a few minutes, though, the coal disintegrated into ash.

In the much cooler aftermath, Jerry saw how his resistance had rendered him as unappreciative and disrespectful of the kids as they were of him. If he led by example, Jerry realized, the whole enterprise would have a different flavor. This realization set off a frenzied round of brainstorming, and within another ten minutes he had a brand-new coaching strategy. The strategy worked. The team's behavior, morale, and performance all improved considerably. Better yet, whenever the kids reverted to their old ways, Jerry no longer took it personally. He was now able to respond to each transgression quickly and creatively, taking the unique needs of each student into full account.

Whenever you talk about emotions, it's as if they're all equal and all good. But some of them are plain inaccurate, even unhealthy, and not just because of conditioning either. Don't you agree that for the purpose of spiritual growth, we often need to rise above certain emotions?

I'm grateful for your invitation to address these issues and will take them one at a time. First, you are absolutely right about emotions sometimes being flat-out wrong without previous conditioning as the cause. But it's my experience that this doesn't happen very often. And to determine if it is happening, we have no other option than to give questionable emotions a full hearing. Usually our verdicts in such cases come much too soon, cut us off from valuable evidence, and end up more about resistance than clear-sighted evaluation. This is akin to punishing a child for misbehavior without learning whether the offense actually occurred. I use the analogy of a child because emotions and children share a tendency toward murky, jumbled communication. It might be nice if emotions were always swift, clear, and to the point, but they aren't.

Second, when you mention that some emotions are unhealthy, I would refine your statement to read, "Prolonged resistance is unhealthy." Unless accompanied by resistance, no emotion appears long enough or frequently enough to cause real harm. When we refer to people in need of anger management, for instance, it's their resistance to anger that's the actual problem. Such people usually need to *stop* trying to manage the experience of anger and instead, finally, just let it happen. Once they can feel their anger fully, without having to act it out upon others, it almost always passes quicker, easier, and minus any social cost. Plus, this process creates a direct line to any core emotion that might lie beneath anger's protective blast (see Kenneth's profile on pages 143–145).

Third, you suggest that some emotions are better or more "spiritual" than others. My own view is that there's a time and place for all of them, but what's more important is that most emotions arise whether we approve of them or not. Therefore, the true test of our virtue is what we do *afterward*. I maintain that the greatest teachers, leaders, healers, and visionaries share an exceptional ability to harmonize with their emotions rather than shoehorn them into a prescribed ideal. Whenever emotions are ranked or denigrated, pushback reigns.

What about the best way to express emotion? Do you have advice about that?

My main advice, to paraphrase one of our earlier mottoes, is "Feel first, speak later." Generally, it's not a good idea to talk about feelings while you're having them, unless with a therapist or similar supporter. As discussed earlier under containment (page 175), doing so tends to decrease connection, increase resistance, and promote inaccurate communication. When you talk about an emotion prior to or during 2 X 2, especially with the parties involved, it's easy to slip into unhelpful criticism, blame, or other forms of accusation. Only when expanded do you have the greatest possibility of saying what you really mean and getting it across in the most fruitful way.

Among the many teachings on effective communication, I'm aware of two that stress emotional connection. The first is Nonviolent Communication, created by Marshall Rosenberg, helps us see the link between our emotions and the needs that engender them, which in turn allows us to formulate skillful spoken requests for our counterparts. The second framework for emotionally connected expression is the Imago Therapy dialogue, created by Harville Hendrix. Here, emphasis is placed upon listening to a counterpart's emotional experience, then validating it fully before otherwise responding.

Still, since there are plenty of times when we don't always have the luxury or ability to wait for expansion before communicating our feelings, it's necessary to have strategies for them too. One such strategy ("drop the rope," introduced on page 165) is to describe only the actual physical sensations you're experiencing. For example, instead of saying something like, "I'm devastated that you forgot my birthday, and it makes me question our relationship," you might say, "I'm feeling sad that you forgot my birthday. My heart is heavy and my throat is tight. Let me have a few minutes to feel all this before we talk about it."

Another strategy for sharing feelings while having them is sticking to one syllable. This is especially helpful for strong emotions that may otherwise lead to regrettable words and for dealing with children or teenagers and their short attention spans. Sometimes just a simple "Owwww!" or "Arrrgh!" is all that's necessary to make sure our emotions are recognized and taken seriously. Plus, if nothing truly serious has occurred, such exclamations can often break the tension and provoke surprising, expansion-inducing amusement.

My life almost always feels chaotic. Sometimes, when I employ 2X 2, the chaos doesn't dissipate, but a calm appears at the center of the storm. Am I doing it right or wrong?

Even though the 2 X 2 process is relevant, appropriate, and helpful for everyone, no two people will apply or experience it in the exact same way. This question describes an unrelenting chaos with a simultaneous expansion at its center, rather than the usual sequence from one to the other. While further 2 X 2 in this situation may bring about more peace and less chaos, it also may not. This could be due to a propensity, conscious or not, for turmoil. In truth, some people thrive on it. So for anyone dealing with such issues, I recommend focusing not on whether you're doing it right or wrong (see assessing on page 65), but instead on what's really true for you. What does your sincere application of the 2 X 2 process teach you about your own unique attributes? In addition, how might this information help you personalize the process?

Often, when I'm 2 X 2-ing about one subject, lots of thoughts and feelings show up about other subjects. Am I doing it right or wrong?

This question highlights how emotions are state dependent, meaning that they often surface in bunches that match the mood of the moment. An angry frame of mind brought about by one situation is likely to produce additional, similar emotions about entirely different subjects. That's because emotions, like life, are messy. If we expect them to follow an orderly or consistent path, via 2 X 2 or otherwise, we'll always be disappointed. But when we do opt for 2 X 2 and encounter a flurry of topics, there's no need to alter our process in any way. For sure this sometimes creates choppy and challenging waters, but they can still be skillfully surfed. Each new topic requires nothing more than a moment of recognition, followed by a resumption of attention on the emotion's physical manifestation.

I come from a long line of people who don't like to feel. It makes us uncomfortable to be so exposed to ourselves and others. I've experimented with the 2 X 2 process but don't get very far. Do you think that's because I'm doing it wrong, or is it possible that some people just aren't wired for deep feeling?

People are, indeed, wired differently. Even if gender, environment, and socialization didn't play roles in the different ways we experience emotion, personality still would. Styles of feeling are as varied as people themselves. The goal of emotional connection, therefore, isn't at all about uniformity. Rather, it's about moving from unconscious habits to free choice, and from self-opposition to self-mastery. This is equally true whether one's lineage is emotionally unbridled, reserved, or somewhere in between.

That said, most of us have a considerable amount of emotional resistance to work through. As a result, the 2 X 2 process does lead us to more feeling, not less. So whenever people define themselves as not particularly emotional, even after a workshop or two, I suggest that they temporarily set aside that self-characterization and seek out a counselor for fine-tuning. Almost always, after putting in that extra effort, they happily revise their original assessment.

COMPENDIUM OF PRINCIPLES AND PRACTICES

Throughout this book, we've covered everything you need to know about emotional connection. You now have the tools to break through any and all self-imposed barriers limiting your fulfillment and success. Admittedly, this simple process is supported by a lot of not-so-simple detail. It can be difficult, therefore, to keep the whole picture in mind. This appendix is designed to help you do that. It provides a quick review of all our main principles and practices. For times requiring further review, relevant page numbers from earlier in the book are also listed.

The 2 X 2 Process

In order to experience emotions directly, **turn your attention to your body.** Whether an emotion appears immediately or is at first blocked by a contraction, **keep your attention on the flow of physical sensation until you reach an expanded state.** The quality of your attention is as important as its placement. **Slow down** your awareness so that emotions are free to arise and clear in their own natural time. **Get microscopic in** your awareness so that emotions can reveal themselves fully, moment-by-moment, beyond the usual labels and abstractions.

Essential Terms

Contraction (56)—a temporary system lockdown, experienced either as tension (fight/flight) or numbness (freeze).

Expansion (60)—a quality of openness and flow. It coexists naturally with positive emotions, but it can also coexist with any emotion. Emotional connection of any kind *produces* expansion.

Addiction/Compulsion (61)—the continuous use of any substance or activity to create disconnection from one's emotions.

Advanced Practices for Challenging Emotions

Breath (44)—Use actual breath and/or your mind's eye. Inhale directly into the stuck bodily sensation. Exhale through that same place, helping to restore inner space and flow.

Posture-movement-sound (45)—Express the internal vibration of an emotion by translating it into these external forms.

Touch (47)—Place a gentle hand on a tense or otherwise uncomfortable physical spot. Keep your hand still or caress the spot lightly.

Direct Inquiry (47)—Let the contraction or emotion speak directly, unmediated by thoughts and concepts. Ask, *If it could speak, what would it say?* Hear the emotion's "voice" to support acceptance of its subjective truth.

Cradling (48)—Cultivate a quality of emotional attention that resembles the spacious, caring way a parent instinctively holds a distressed infant.

Mental Detachment (52)—Maintain an even-keeled awareness of thoughts, beliefs, and stories that arise while practicing 2 X 2.

Rather than pushing them away or getting lost in them, simply note their presence, along with any immediate response they produce, and then return your focus to emotional flow.

Obstacles to Emotional Connection

Analyzing (62)—Trying to figure out *why* an emotion is occurring rather than experiencing it directly.

Judging (64)—Looking for *what's wrong* with an emotion—or with you for having it—rather than continuing to feel.

Assessing (65) –Getting lost in an evaluation of your process, which usually takes the form or an obsessive quest to "do it right."

Bargaining (65)—Placing any preset limits or conditions on emotional connection, whether in regard to duration, depth, or outcome.

Using Emotional Connection to Get Unstuck

Find the Flinch (chapter 6)—Identify the aspect of moving forward with your vision that causes you to pull up short.

Cut to the Chase (chapter 7)—Discover your worst-case scenario in moving forward, and determine how that outcome would make you feel.

Weather the Storm (chapter 8)—Use all of your creative power to imagine that outcome as a reality, then surf the whole cascade of emotions that comes with it.

Repeat as Necessary (chapter 9)—Apply the above course of action whenever you get stuck again in pursuit of your goal, regarding both the same emotions and any possible new ones.

Understand the Triune Brain (84)—This working model of your mind supports the above method for getting unstuck. It presents the brain's three main systems—primitive, limbic, neocortex—in order of their evolutionary development. Following the same order in any difficult situation is the fastest, easiest way to restore peak function. In other words, first release whatever contraction is present (primitive brain). Next, feel all the emotions present (limbic system). Then, and only then, employ creative, abstract reasoning (neocortex). Attempting to achieve peak function in any other order, by contrast, foments confusion and repression.

22 Key Refinements

Reconstructed Walk–through (103)—To reveal and release the emotional "motor" of a compulsion, focus on a recent and/or intense version of the usual compulsive episode. Replay it in your mind's eye in superslow motion with special attention to your bodily state at each micromoment. Once you zero in on the emotions that usually get glossed over, stay with them till the onset of expansion.

Images and Personas (104)—Recognize that emotions often arise with corresponding internal images. Welcome these images as pathways to deeper understanding and release. Stay especially attuned to images of yourself at very young ages, experiencing related challenges to whatever you face currently.

Done-deal Delay (109)—When the trip wire goes off in your brain to engage in compulsive activity, experiment with brief delays in assenting to that habitual decision. Increase the delay slowly and incrementally, using the 2 X 2 process to attend to all the contraction and emotion that inevitably results. Notice, as the underlying emotions receive this new attention, how the intensity of the compulsive response begins to diminish.

Self-acceptance (109)—In asserting our willpower to change personal behavior, one part of us inevitably fights against another. In such a case, the losing side always exacts some kind of revenge. This is referred to as **pushback**, and it leads to a new, unhealthy equilibrium even if the originally desired change has occurred. To avoid this, practice self-acceptance, which means connecting emotionally to all parts of you, even the ones you don't want. Self-acceptance allows you to move from an either/or perspective to one of **both/and**.

The No-fail Zone (112)—If you attempt to practice the 2 X 2 process and don't succeed, consider this not a failure but a learning opportunity. Pay close attention to what shut you down, thereby allowing you to be more prepared for it the next time. This practice is a form of self-acceptance vital for clearing the most scary and entrenched emotions.

Pinpointing (113)—Emotional connection can only proceed as quickly and fully as the most tentative part of you can go. When you dive in too fast, significant pushback results. To pinpoint means breaking down your experience of a difficult emotion into tiny, manageable amounts. For best effect, cultivate an honest, patient, consistent awareness of your limits.

The Adrenaline Factor (117)—A rush of adrenaline in connection with any repetitive activity is a sure indicator of emotional repression. Think of it as a giant stop sign, and then use the ensuing pause to unravel the urge's emotional content.

Stand in the Fire (121)—Compulsions are both a call for attention and a kind of lie. They trick us into thinking that satisfying the current desire will lead to fulfillment. The truth is that underneath every compulsion is a deeper need for emotional connection. Sometimes in order to encourage that connection, it's helpful to stand in the fire of your compulsion. This means focusing on one or more of the worst ways the behavior impacts your life. The goal isn't to punish yourself, but instead to burn away your compulsive trance.

The Fork in the Road (130)—Before making important decisions, assess the degree of resistance present in each possible choice. Only when you've used the 2 X 2 process to render all paths resistance free can you be confident in both the decision-making process and the decision itself.

Tactical Empathy (132)—Developing the ability to resonate with your own emotions also makes it possible to resonate with other people's emotions. Tactical empathy means employing such resonance with partners and groups, while simultaneously remaining connected to yourself, to serve the highest good of all.

The Emotional Audit (134)—Emotions and resistance to them play dominant roles in almost every group. This dominance is usually unconscious and rarely understood. An emotional audit reveals a group's general ethos, as well as the way emotions are approached, understood, valued, shared, and processed. There is no one best way to perform such an audit. Choose a method for your group that's likeliest to produce the greatest degree of honesty and cooperation.

Mutability (137)—The 2 X 2 process illuminates the way emotions shift fluidly from one to another, both moment by moment and over time. In addition, multiple emotions often arise about a single topic. This is totally natural. As long as you meet all such mutability with a both/and orientation, it will enrich your emotional connection rather than impede it.

Exaggeration (141)—When advanced practices for emotional connection don't lead to sufficient feeling and expansion, exaggeration is the next option. Dramatize and express the emotion far beyond its actual intensity. Often this breaks the logjam, allowing you to quickly resume ordinary 2 X 2 with the emotion in its unexaggerated state.

Emotional Association (142)—While exaggeration is an experiential way to get unstuck, emotional association is its mental correlate. Here, simply ask yourself, *When have I felt this way before?* Let the past events that surface in response to this inquiry both illuminate and add "juice" to your current attempt at connection. If the above question doesn't do the trick, also try asking, *What similar situations have I experienced before?*

Working with Physical Pain (145)—Sometimes physical pain is somaticized, meaning that it's been created as a result of resisted, unconscious emotion. In addressing any ache or pain that is as yet undiagnosed, connect to it for at least five minutes with the 2 X 2 process. If an emotion is indeed the cause, this will allow it to surface and release, eliminating most or even all of the pain. When an emotion isn't the cause, attending to bodily complaints in this way still reveals how you feel *about* the pain. It also creates the best internal environment to ease discomfort of any type or origin.

Protective vs. Core Emotions (146)—Emotions often arise to screen us from other more challenging emotions. These emotions are part of our primitive brain's defensive mechanism. Maintaining a sustained connection with protective emotions enables core ones to surface and clear. Until they do, such protective-core patterns remain stubbornly fixed.

Proportional Response (152)—Life inevitably presents situations where complete emotional connection or complete emotional repression isn't optimal. For these middle-ground situations, use the practice of proportional response, connecting with just the right amount of emotion to keep you sufficiently present and expanded for the task at hand. Once the current challenge has passed, find the soonest possible time to employ the 2 X 2 process full force.

Button Power (157)—The people and situations that push our buttons, while definitely unpleasant, also provide the greatest possibility for emotional breakthrough. Keep a keen eye out for whatever pushes your own buttons both frequently and intensely. Train yourself, for maximum effect, to apply the 2 X 2 process right in the heat of the moment.

Drop the Rope (165)—When two people are in resistance, it's all too easy for conflicts to escalate. Just one person, however, has the power to break this cycle. As soon as you become aware that you're in such a tug-of-war, drop the rope, using these steps: (1) find your physical contraction; (2) describe the sensations of that contraction to your counterpart; (3) pause the discussion and separate; (4) use 2 X 2 until expansion occurs; and (5) resume the discussion, resistance free.

Positive Boundaries (168)—A positive boundary is a nondefensive approach to self-protection that allows you to feel both safe and expansive at the same time. To create one, connect to the state of well-being within yourself, and then use your mind's eye to imagine it extending beyond your physical body. Stretch your boundary to a distance at which usually hurtful comments and behaviors no longer make a serious dent. With practice, you'll need to stretch it less and less.

Containment (173)—Most emotions compel us to talk about them, and we often do so long before a conversation can actually produce a beneficial result. Containment, therefore, is an indispensable tool. As a general rule, don't talk about an emotion until you've connected with it directly for a significant amount of time. If possible, wait until you're become fully expanded.

Seeing through Projection (177)—When projecting, we misplace our thoughts, feelings, or interpretations about one person upon another. Resisted emotion is almost always the cause, and emotional connection is almost always the solution. There are three reliable indicators that you may be projecting in a given situation: (1) physical contraction; (2) an excessive reaction; and (3) persistent thoughts about a similar event from the past. To spot possible projection in other people, look for the presence of indicators two and three above. In addition, if you ask people directly whether they might be projecting, a highly charged response provides another affirmative sign.

Additional Tools

Distinguishing between Soft and Hard Resistance (162)—Soft resistance is a temporary, easily surmountable inclination not to feel. Hard resistance is a recognition that the time is definitely not right for emotional connection. When you can't tell which you're experiencing, give the 2 X 2 process another full minute. At that point, if your connection has been genuine, any remaining resistance is more than likely hard.

Screen Door (203)—If you want to avoid feeling the emotions of those around you and don't want to erect a positive boundary, instead imagine yourself as a screen door. Regard all emotions you experience as breezes blowing through the screen. Emotions that "stick" are yours to feel, and all the rest will pass right through.

Proportional Vulnerability (204)—People vary widely in their openness to the emotions of others. It makes good sense, therefore, to assess every person and social situation in this light. Reveal only as much of your emotions as will likely be welcome. When in doubt, proceed with caution, recalibrating your vulnerability often to meet current conditions.

Handling your Inner Two-year-old (209)—Most of us have a lively internal naysayer stuck forever in the "terrible twos," who raises a ruckus in regard to many of our necessary activities. Meet your own naysayer with a both/and perspective, letting it have a complete say. This approach reveals that the goal of most tantrums is to be heard, not to actually thwart your actions. Once you give your inner two-year-old the chance to stomp around and protest, it usually settles right down.

How Not to Take Things Personally (211–212)—Consider people and their behaviors to be natural, unavoidable parts of the world around you. Birds fly, fish swim, people hurt your feelings. When you accept this as a fact and not a problem, it gives you the opportunity to detach your attention from the cause of an upset and shift it to the physical result. Once you're surfing your own emotions, the original hurt will quickly lose its sting. This frees you to address the overall situation and the offending party with a much lighter touch.

One-syllable Communication (215)—Many emotions need to be expressed simply as raw energy. When this happens, words can get in the way and end up causing all kinds of additional, unnecessary problems. In place of words, a groan, growl, "Ow!" or "Hey!" often gets your point across safely and quickly. Sometimes, such one-syllable utterances even leaven the situation with humor.

GRATITUDE

Along the journey from concept to publication, this book has been graced by many angels. First came Dawn Raffel and Amy Gross at *O, The Oprah Magazine,* who helped me shape the material in article form. Next came Oprah Winfrey herself, who selected the article for her *Live Your Best Life* anthology. My ever-enthusiastic agent, Eileen Cope, guided me in nurturing the project into a book and finding it the best possible home. Gideon Weil, my editor, provided clear, spot-on assistance in maximizing the manuscript's potential. Jan Weed, Alison Petersen, and the whole HarperOne team attended to each detail with great care in the final stages of production.

The first words for *One Thing* came to me on a teaching stint at the Esalen Institute. In the cottage constructed for the late Fritz Perls, I gained strength from his wizardly persona, danced a lot, and wrote a little. Back home, during the bulk of the writing, my always-patient bride, Traci, heeded every single call for late-night paragraph review. Her intuitive responses often led to crucial additions of dimension and texture. As deadlines loomed and health waned, it was beloved Hazel who would inevitably uplift me with a round of jump-offs or fly-highs.

When Esmeralda, Jezebel, and Lothario showed up, inspiration was never far behind. Then came Aria Belle, at first with an endless wail and then a heart-melting grin. She brought me steady focus even in the midst of great trials. Throughout those trials, Bob Cushnir, and Sherrie and Bob Stahl provided indispensable support. So, too, did Kelli and Tom Thomsen, and Terry Patten. Then, when the book needed a final nudge toward its widest possible audience, Rachel Dyer was a kind, incisive sage.

I'm also extraordinarily grateful to the countless students and teachers who have sat in session with me since I began developing this material many years ago. You're all here somewhere, whether in the text itself or between the lines. It's you, with your courageous, vulnerable, openhearted sharing, who brought these pages to life.

From my Jewish heritage comes the word "shalom," meaning hello, good-bye, and peace. From the Hindu tradition comes the word "Namaste," meaning "the Spirit in me recognizes and honors the Spirit in you." At the end of every workshop I combine these two words in joyful parting. Now, to everyone who aided this book, and to its readers as well, I'd like to do the same. And so, I say to you all . . . *Shalomaste.*

STAYING CONNECTED

Any and all communication from readers of this book is encouraged and appreciated. To share your questions, "yeah, buts," comments, stories, and reflections about emotional connection, please e-mail me directly at rc@emotionalconnection.org.

I'm especially interested in hearing from you if the principles and practices in the book aren't working to full effect in your own life or organization. All e-mails sent to the above address are confidential, and I'm the only person who reads them. I'll do my very best to respond quickly and to offer relevant, helpful suggestions.

To learn about scheduling emotional-connection keynotes and trainings, please visit:

www.emotionalconnection.org.

This Web site is also where you can learn about workshops, retreats, counseling by phone, and how to become a certified emotional connection instructor.